The Recent Topics in Genetic Polymorphisms

Edited by Mahmut Çalışkan, Osman Erol and Gül Cevahir Öz

Published in London, United Kingdom

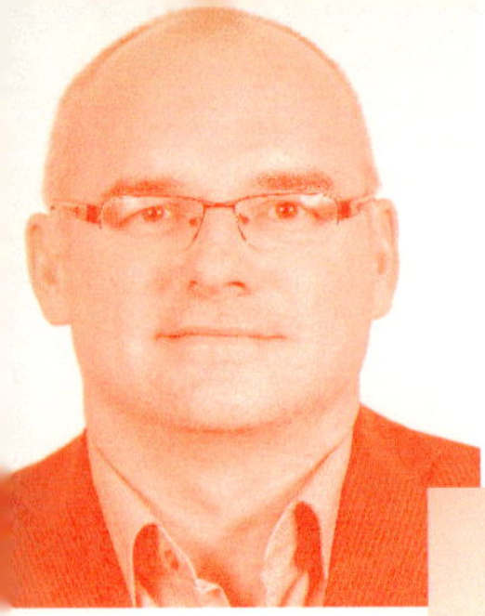
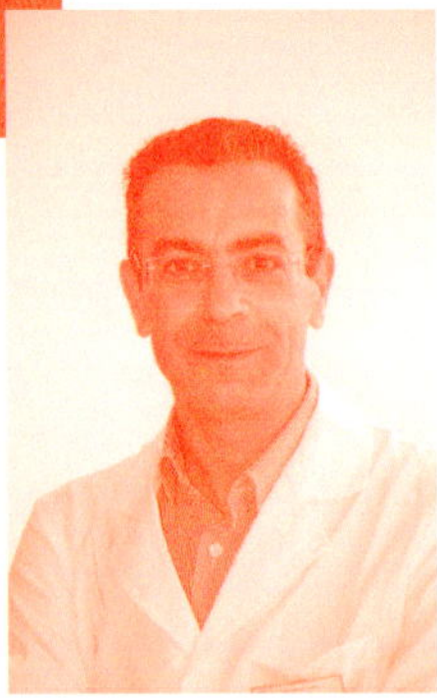
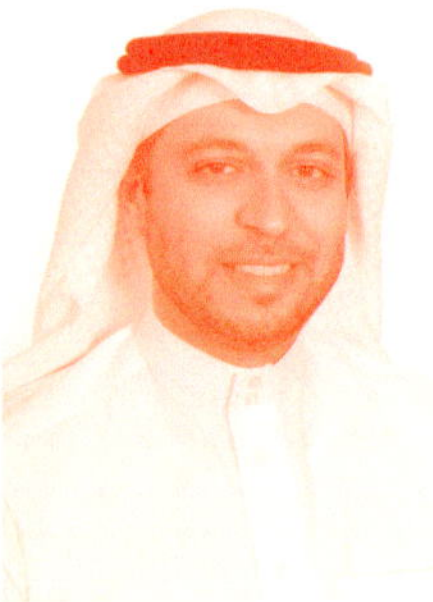
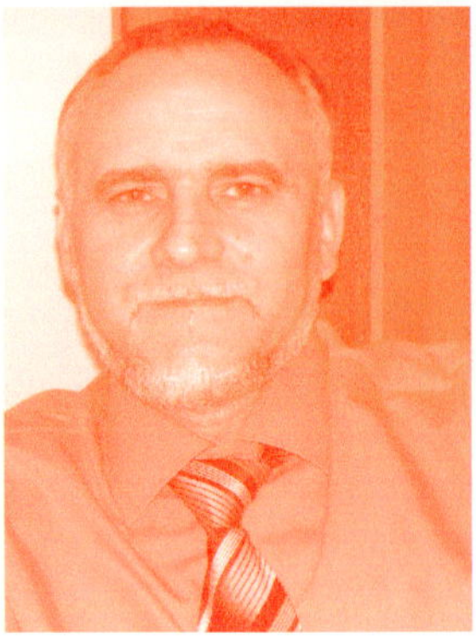
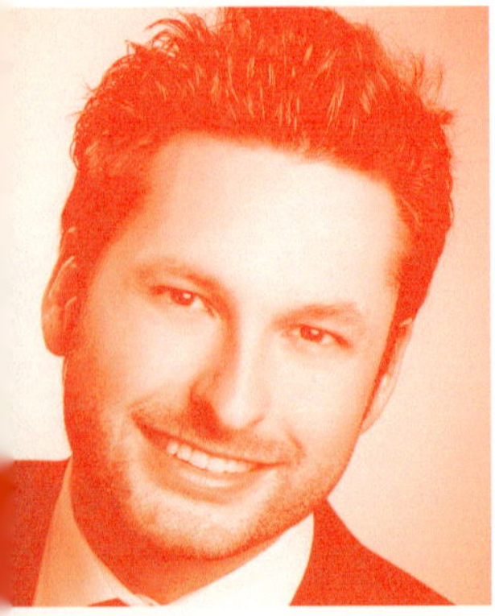
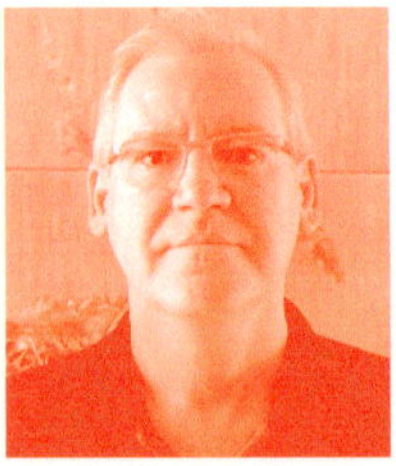
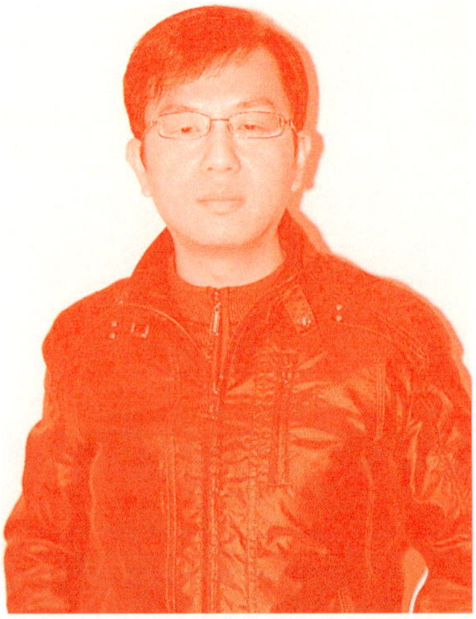

IntechOpen

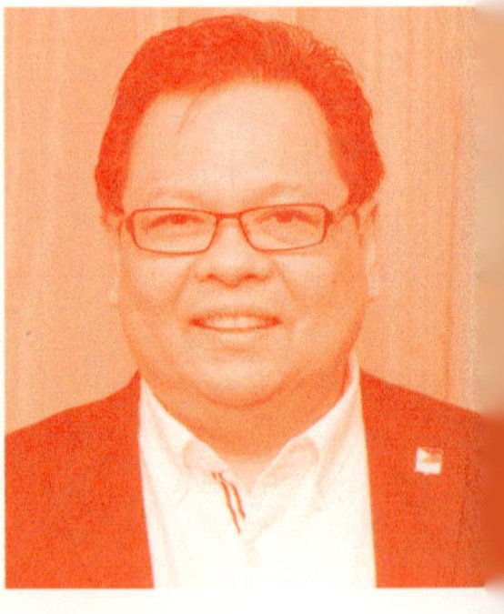
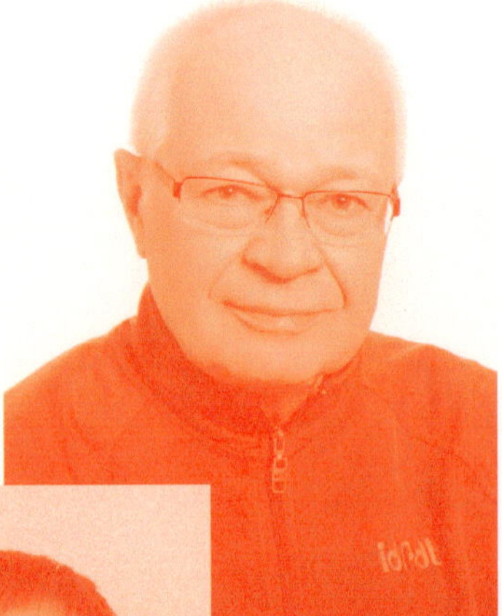
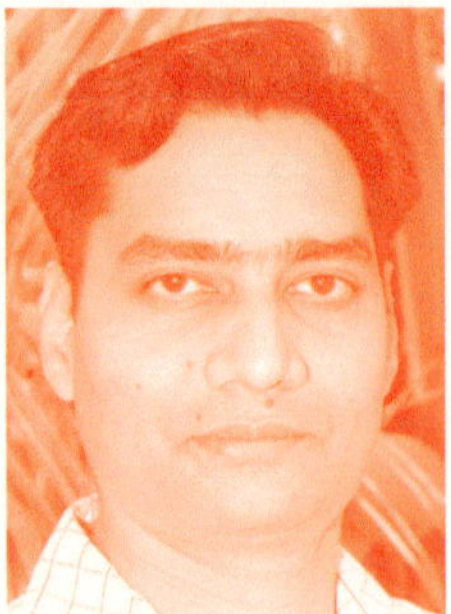
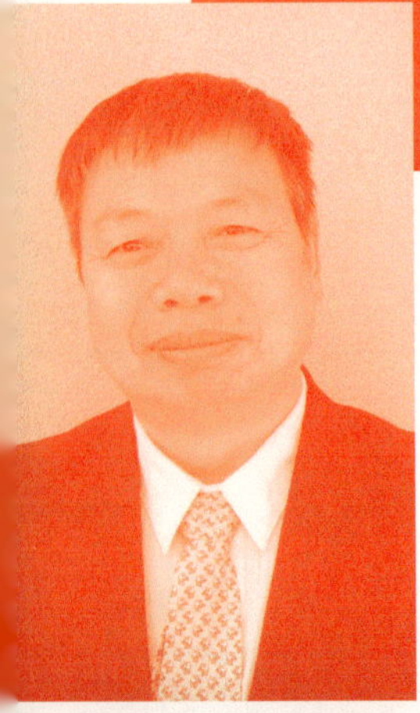
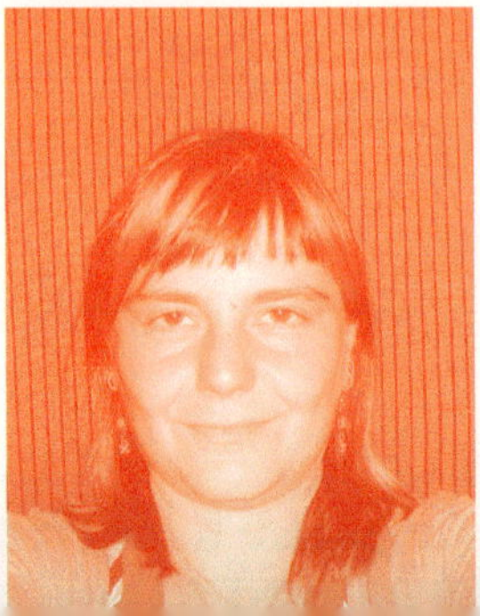
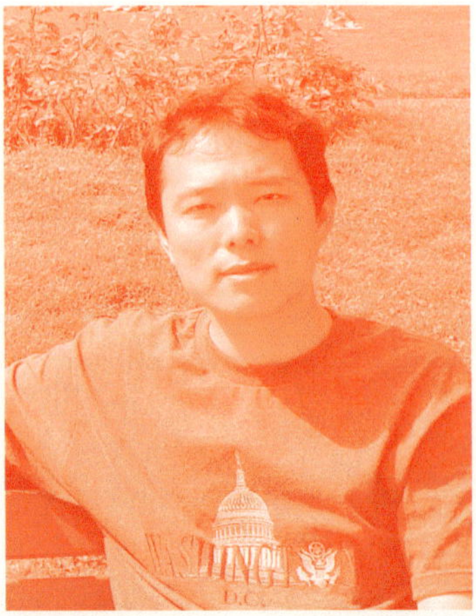

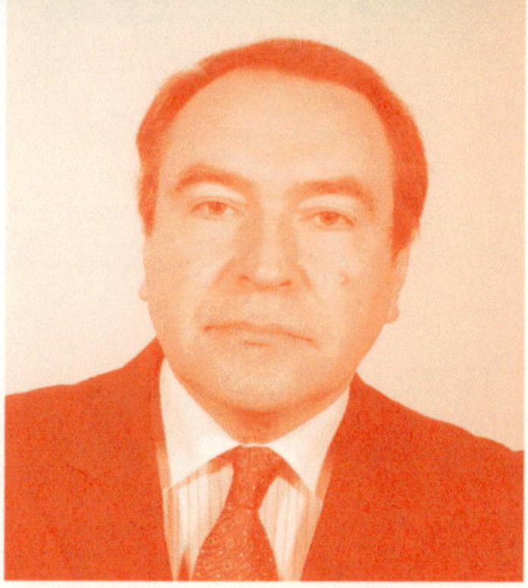
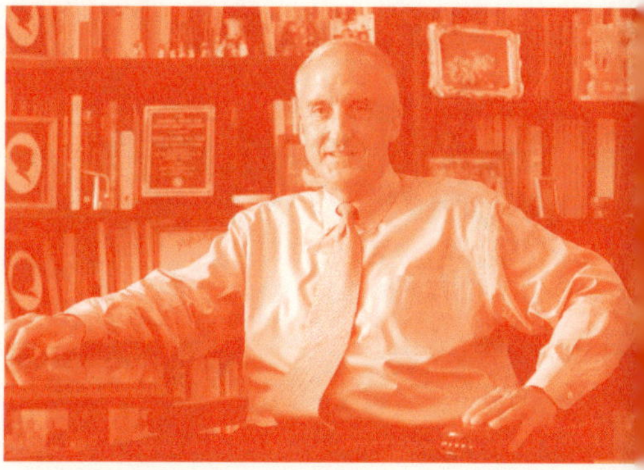
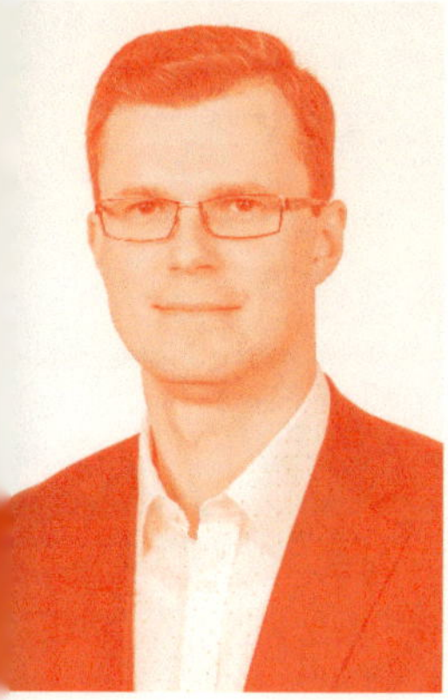
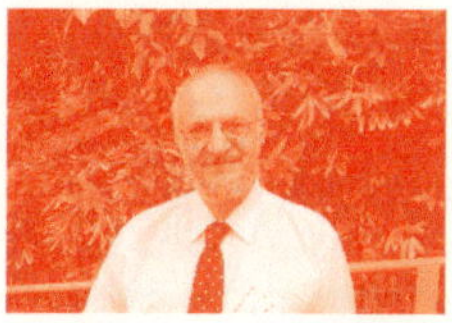
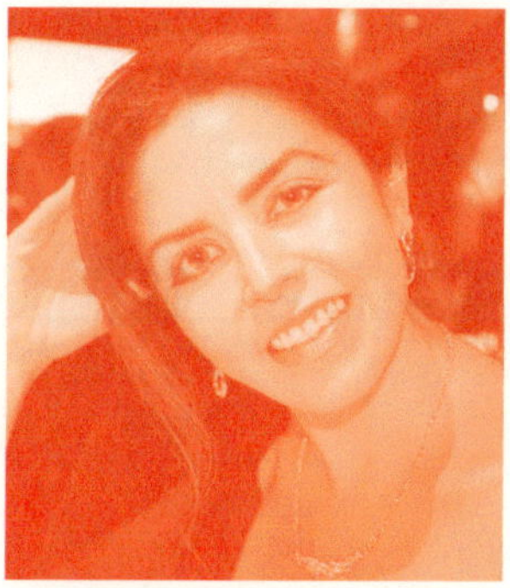

Supporting open minds since 2005

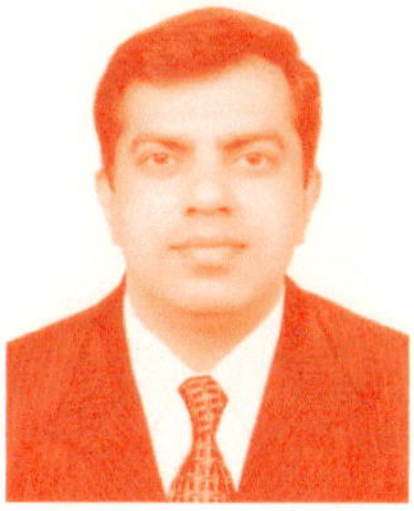
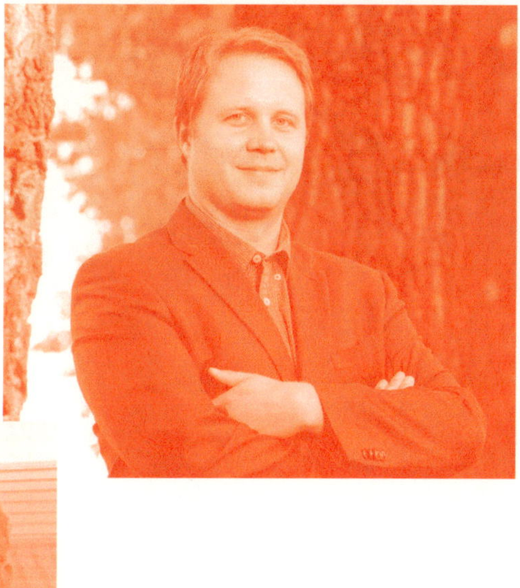
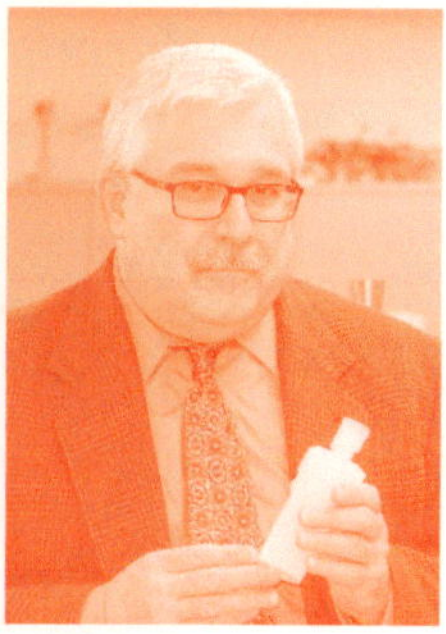
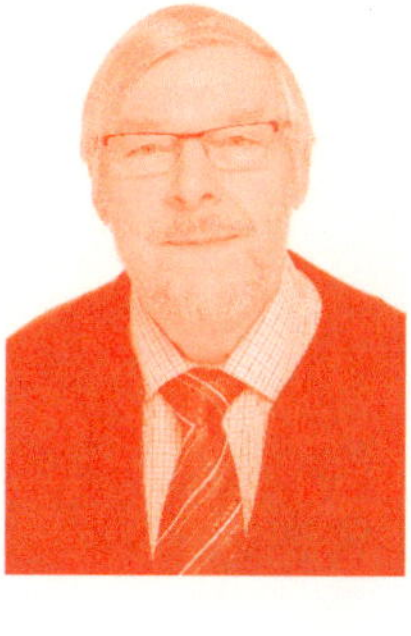
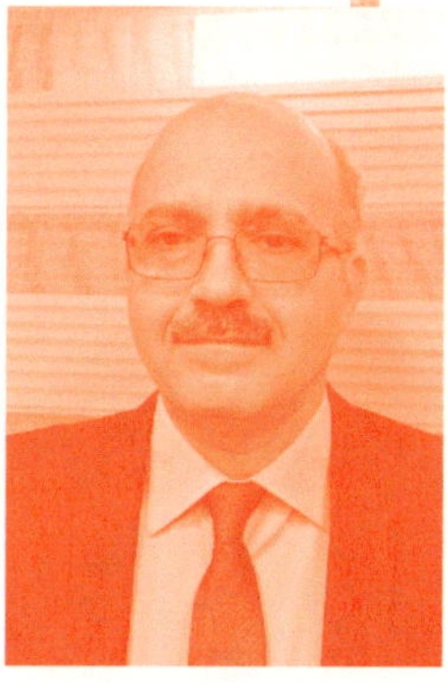
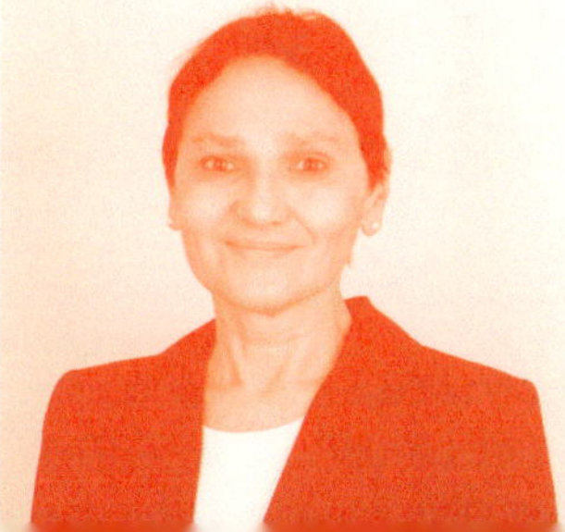
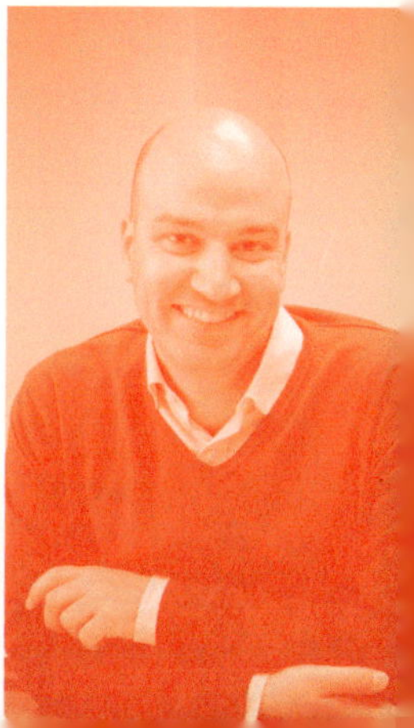

The Recent Topics in Genetic Polymorphisms
http://dx.doi.org/10.5772/intechopen.77777
Edited by Mahmut Çalışkan, Osman Erol and Gül Cevahir Öz

Contributors
Muhammad Tarek Abdel Ghafar, Pieranna Chiarella, Pasquale Capone, Renata Sisto, Dhafer Al-Koofee, Shaden Hasan, Subodh Jain, Sapna Sedha, Meeta Mishra, Misbahul Arfin, Ghaleb Bin Huraib, Abdulrahman Al-Asmari, Fahad Al- Harthi, Ewa Dudzińska, Hande Morgil, Işıl Tulum, Yusuf Can Gercek

First published in London, United Kingdom, 2020 by IntechOpen
IntechOpen is the global imprint of INTECHOPEN LIMITED, registered in England and Wales, registration number: 11086078, 7th floor, 10 Lower Thames Street, London, EC3R 6AF, United Kingdom
Printed in Croatia

British Library Cataloguing-in-Publication Data
A catalogue record for this book is available from the British Library

Additional hard and PDF copies can be obtained from orders@intechopen.com

The Recent Topics in Genetic Polymorphisms
Edited by Mahmut Çalışkan, Osman Erol and Gül Cevahir Öz
p. cm.
Print ISBN 978-1-78985-891-4
Online ISBN 978-1-78985-892-1
eBook (PDF) ISBN 978-1-78984-622-5

For EU product safety concerns:
IN TECH d.o.o., Prolaz Marije Krucifikse Kozulić 3, 51000 Rijeka, Croatia, info@intechopen.com or visit our website at intechopen.com.

Meet the editors

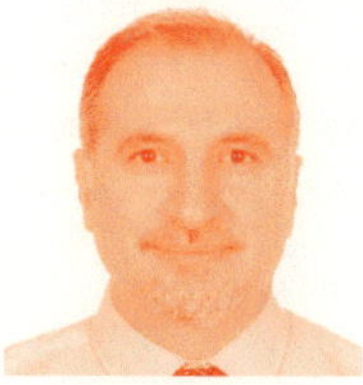

Mahmut Çalışkan is a professor of genetics and molecular biology in the Department of Biology at Istanbul University in Turkey. He obtained his first degree, BSc, from the Middle East Technical University, Ankara and attended the University of Leeds, Department of Genetics, England for his PhD. His main research areas include the role of germin gene products during early plant development and the characterization and biotechnological use of halophilic archaea.

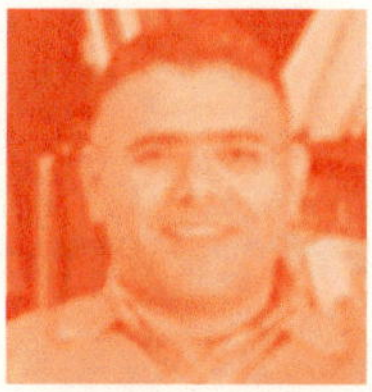

Osman Erol was born in 1974. After completing his BSc degree from the Istanbul University, he received his MSc degree in 1999 and his PhD in 2004. His specialty is the Iridaceae family, Ixioideae subfamily. He is currently working on saffron and its relatives. Osman Erol is an associate professor at Istanbul University Science Faculty.

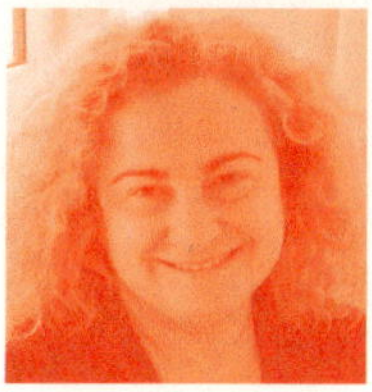

Gül Cevahir Öz is a professor in the Department of Biology at Istanbul University. She received her PhD in plant physiology from Istanbul University in 1997. Her present interests include starch synthesis, especially the mechanism of ADP-glucose phyrophosphorylase, the role of hormones in plant development, biochemical and molecular mechanisms of plant tolerance to abiotic stress, and plant biotechnology.

Contents

Preface

Ever since human beings adopted a diverse way of life on earth, they have continuously attempted to improve on what they found in nature including all kinds of living beings. Once they came to understand that living beings' characteristics are inherited and genetic richness is an advantage against changing environmental conditions, they have developed new strategies to reveal and conserve the genetic diversity in living beings. The main evolutionary mechanisms such as mutation, natural selection, and genetic drift have produced a vast variation of organisms that ended in the formation of many well-defined breeds with different levels of performance. The knowledge of genetic polymorphism and process that underlie the origins and maintenance of the organisms have crucial importance in providing critical insights into the structure and dynamics of living populations. Genetic polymorphism is essential for populations to evolve and cope with environmental changes, new diseases, and pest epidemics. Genetic polymorphisms also provide the opportunity for tracing the history of populations, species, and their ancestors. Therefore, the assessment of genetic variation in species and among populations is important for conservation of genetic resources. Detailed knowledge of genetic variation within and among different breeds is very important for understanding and improving traits of economic importance. Hence, the future improvement is dependent on genetic variation present within breeds and between breed variation.

Over the last few decades there have been dramatic advances in molecular genetics and these developments have provided scientists involved in the conservation and improvement of genetic resources with a range of new techniques for their research. Nowadays techniques are available to determine changes at the DNA level in all kinds of organisms. Differences in gene sequences can be directly observed and described with a degree of precision previously impossible to achieve. Many of the techniques that have been developed have already been used to study the extent and distribution of changes in gene-pool and to investigate evolutionary and taxonomic relationships. With the development of the polymerase chain reaction (PCR) based techniques, in particular, numerous molecular technologies have been, and still are being, developed, which can be used for the detection, characterization, and evaluation of genetic changes in populations. These techniques can be chosen on the basis of how they display genetic differences, the type of data that they produce, the taxonomic levels at which they can be most appropriately applied, and their technical and financial requirements.

The aim of this book is to present the current knowledge of genetic polymorphisms by including the works of some of the scientists engaged in the production of new information used to reveal genetic polymorphisms, often from very different perspectives. Chapters presented in the book demonstrate the future benefit of molecular markers including SNPs in many studies retaining the genetic polymorphisms. In the book, the genetic polymorphism studies that are carried out on different kinds of organisms at the DNA level or gene expression level are particularly important to evaluate the process of genetic polymorphisms.

The purpose of the current book is to provide a glimpse into the dynamic process of genetic polymorphism by presenting valuable research. I would like to express my deepest gratitude to all authors who contributed to this book by sharing their valuable works with us. This book should prove useful to students, researchers, and experts in the area of molecular genetics.

Dr. Mahmut Çalişkan
Professor,
İstanbul University Faculty of Sciences,
Biology Department Biotechnology Division,
Istanbul, Turkey

Dr. Osman Erol
Professor,
Istanbul University,
Turkey

Dr. Gül Cevahir Öz
Professor,
Department of Biology at Istanbul University,
Turkey

Chapter 1

Genetic Polymorphisms

Dhafer A.F. Al-Koofee and Shaden M.H. Mubarak

Abstract

It is amazing to know that around 99.9% of the individuals genome among persons is alike, and only 0.1% of it differs in chromosome. This variance is accountable for the diversity in phenotypes and receptiveness of them to environmental effects. DNA variants are happening in numerous formulas. Mutations might be definite as order variants which happen in less than 1% of the populace, whereas the extra prevalent variant is identified as polymorphisms. More than 1% of the greatest public hereditary variants are known as single nucleotide polymorphisms (SNPs). In human genome, SNPs considered as plentiful figure of genetic variation, and their importance in contribution to many disease, drug efficacy, and side effects in addition to may represent a prophylaxis. SNPs represent a specific location at which more than one nucleotide is established and only two alleles at a SNP locus. More than 100 million SNPs have been recognized in human, in average each 300 nucleotide on usual. The gene which has more than one allele is a normal result of SNP. SNPs are not restricted to coding sequence, but may be associated with non-coding region. Many techniques are used to analyze SNPs and involve two phases, one for allele recognition and another for detection.

Keywords: SNP, allele frequency, point mutation, VNP, chromosome, gender, gene, VNTR, CNV, STR

1. Introduction

Genetics terms returns to origin from Greek genetikos meaning "genitive," which in turn derives from genesis meaning "origin" [1, 2]. Genetics in general is a branch of biology related to survey of genes, genetic variation, and even heredity in living systems [3–5]. The study of inheritance pattern that influences genes on human nature and occurs in human beings is called human genetics. Human genetics represents an original aspect that encompasses a variety of overlapping fields like the structure of gene and organization; the study of mutation detection; genetic mapping and linkage analysis; molecular diagnostics; gene expression; cytogenetics assessment; biomedical genetics; disease association studies; tumorigenesis of molecular levels; developmental genetics; and genetic epidemiology, in addition to genetics of complex disease [6, 7]. In general, genes can be considered as a key of most human inherited lesions. So, the benefit study of human genetics can be helpful to answer many questions concerning human diseases and invent effective drugs [8]. The passing of a certain genes from parents to offspring by biological process is called heredity. Each baby carries genes from their biological parents and some of these genes express particular trait or lesion [9]. Various traits may be physical like color of eyes, hair, skin, and other phenotypic matter. In other direction, some genes may play a key role in the risk of certain disorders and increase incidence of disease, or prophylaxis from it [10]. Several disorders occur and arise from multiple factors such as genetic, lifestyle, and environmental [11]. Many previous studies revealed facts for the hereditability of main neuropsychiatric disorders, for example, depression, bipolar disorder, and schizophrenia [12, 13]. In all these behavioral disorders, a specific genetic fault is transported from parents to children and will enhance a progeny susceptibility risk of inheriting a specific disorder [11, 12, 14, 15].

Neurological and mental diseases cannot be related to genetics science alone, so it is significant to seek implicated one's genetic composition material that possibly affects various direction of human behavior [16]. The relationship between genes and behavior leads to development of highly prevalent responses and disorders throughout a new biological factors. About 30–50% of the risk for anxiety and depression is genetic, while the other 50–70% of the risk may be attributed to environmental factors, such as substance use, stress, diet, and childhood experiences [17]. A comparison between genetic and environmental factors, demonstrated about 30–50% of the risk for anxiety and depression and 50–70% of substance uses, stress, and diet, respectively [17, 18].

2. Genes in the cell

Not each living cell of the human body have nucleus. Skin, hair, and red blood cells contain no nucleus [19, 20]. Nucleus contains a genetic material that is responsible for information. Half of these information of the genetic materials come from each parent [20].

2.1 Chromosome

All nuclei of human cell contain 23 pairs of small thread-like structures called chromosomes. Genes are localized within these 23 pairs chromosomes. About 23 out of 46 chromosomes come from the father and others like them come from the mother [21]. These chromosomes contain genes and some of them carry thousands of important genes while some carry only a few [22]. In addition to these, genes are made up of a chemical substance named deoxyribonucleic acid (DNA). The chromosomes are very long thread strands of DNA, coiled up tightly and compacted [23].

Along every chromosome, there is a constriction point called centromere, the numbering and divided packages of chromosome started from it [24]. The centromere separates the chromosome into two arms: long called "q arm" and short called "p arm" as in **Figure 1**. Chromosomes are numbered from 1 to 22 in both sexes and called autosomes, while the last one remaining take letters X and Y which are responsible for the gender. In female, X chromosome is duplicated, whereas Y chromosome is combined with X chromosome in male [24, 25] (**Figures 2** and **3**).

2.2 Nitrogenous bases

The nitrogenous bases are organic molecule with a nitrogen atom that bears chemical prosperities of a base and involves four letters in addition to fifth letter used in ribonucleic acid (RNA), and classified into two main compounds: pyrimidine cytosine (C), thymine (T), and uracil (U); and purine guanine (G) and adenine (A), respectively [27]. They were arranged in unique position in genes, which makes up combinations with permutations and combinations. It is worth mentioning (AT and GC) that bases pair is always found together, and there are different sequences

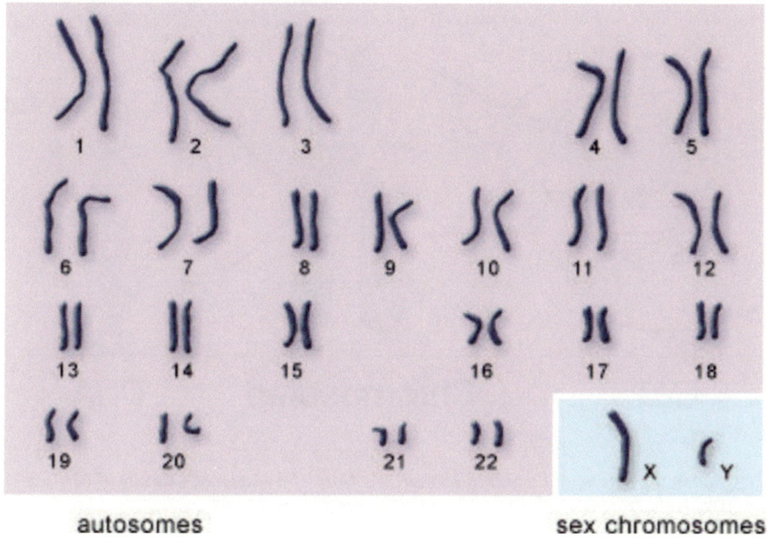

Figure 1.
Autosomes and sex chromosomes of Homo sapiens from US National Library of Medicine, National Institutes of Health, Department of Health & Human Services. June 4, 2012.

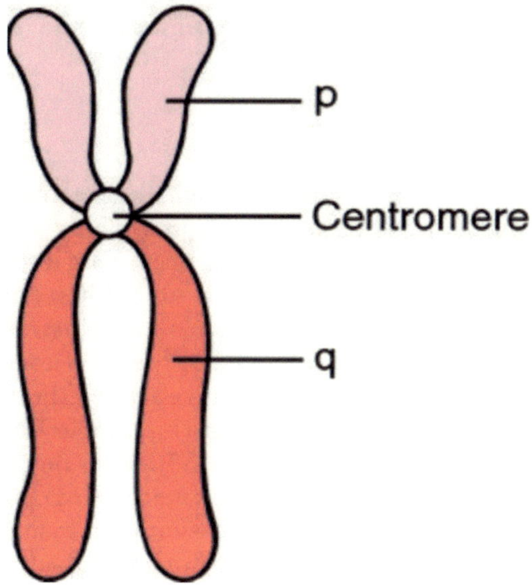

Figure 2.
Chromosome structure explained long and short arms [26].

of bases pairs in DNA coded messages [28]. These bases are part of DNA, and constitute a language when arranged together acting as a guide telling cells what need to do such as growing, division, maturity, and variety functions [29].

2.3 Gender

Both gender have 46 paired chromosomes (44 autosomes), numbered from 1 to 22 chromosome pairs according to size, chromosome number 1 being the biggest one. In addition to autosomes, there are other two copies of sex chromosomes X and Y responsible for determination of gender. In female, two copies of X chromosome

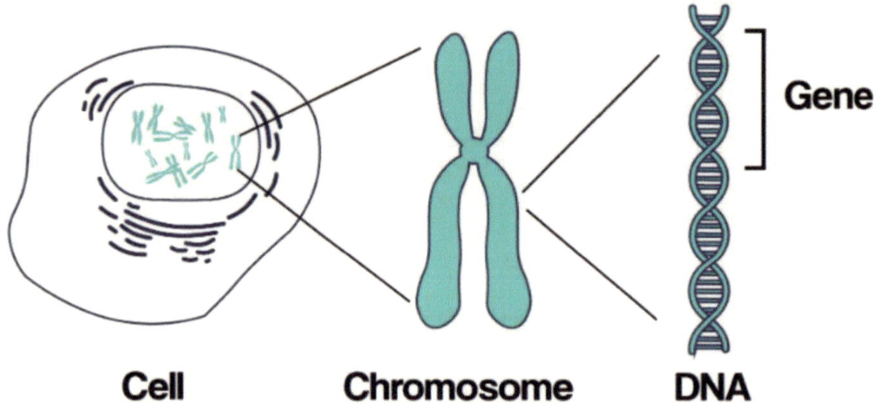

Figure 3.
Distribution of gene in the chromosome within human cell from U S National Library of Medicine, National Institutes of Health, Department of Health & Human Services. June 4, 2012.

are present, while in male, one X copy and one Y copy in their body cells. In female, 22 autosomes paired chromosomes in addition to X sex chromosome present in the egg cells, while in male, the same number of chromosomes are present and the difference only X or Y chromosome in their sperm cells. The combination egg with sperm gives 46 chromosomes regarding the sex chromosome (XY in male and XX in female babies) [30, 31].

2.4 Human genes and genetics

The whole DNA in the cell makes a genome which contains both the exon (coding regions) and intron (non-coding region) that represent large sequences that do not encode any protein and their function is exactly not known yet [32, 33]. In genome, the gene is a basic biological functional unit of heredity that contributes to phenotype/function. A segment of DNA that encodes instruction is needed for a certain protein or enzyme. In other side, a lot of genes do not encode any protein. Only a fraction of DNA of the gene in the cell is expressed through transcription process that involves copy of chemical bases into messenger RNA (mRNA) in order to produce protein according to central dogma [33]. After that it will be translated by using ribosomes organelles, and mRNA migrates toward cytoplasm from nucleus to create polypeptide that folds in a certain configuration to make the protein. A range of human genes are between hundred to more than two millions of nitrogen bases. About 20,000–25,000 genes are located on the 23 pairs of chromosomes within nucleus according to human genome project [34]. The human genome project completed officially in April 2003, and only 12,800 genes and numerous other genes have been well mapped to loci on each of the chromosomes. On the other hand, the correct number of human gene is still unknown [35, 36].

In human being, any individual has two copies from each gene, one copy comes from father and second copy comes from mother [32]. In all people, most genes are similar, excluding small number of genes that are little a bit diverse between people (<1%). The alternative form of a gene that occurs at the same locus on homologous chromosomes called allele bears a small variation in their DNA sequences and participates to every person's single physical features. A single allele for each gene is inherited from each parent (e.g., at a locus for hair or eye color and blood type). About 2% only of genome represent the DNA in genes and full information is stored in a database that is publicly accessible [37].

2.5 Inherit characteristics

Genes are considered as building blocks of inheritance [38]. The traits pass from parents to their offspring and are controlled by some genes; these are carried out by either sexual or asexual reproduction [39]. The genetic information and characteristics are acquired in the progeny cells from their natural parents. However, most of them are affected by mixing the environmental effect and genes. Many traits are observed simply like tongue rolling, dimples, freckles, hands clasping, etc. [40].

2.6 Dominant, recessive, and co-dominant genes

The cell works via coded messages that send from both alleles of genes that involved in every set of chromosomes. Some of these genes appear dominant more than other in works [41]. The dominant occurs when one allele of gene is dominant, while the recessive appears in opposite to dominant within the pair. However, there is present other situation neither dominant nor recessive called homozygous [32]. Homozygous is an equal weight carrier combination of each allele in the gene pair and demonstrates phenotypic and physical characteristics between them [42].

2.7 The genetic keys

The genetic information that endures on the genes order to produce specific protein will be converted to "switched on" position in a few specific specialized cells, and at the same time, other genes may be "switched off" position [43]. Cells differ in differentiation, so genes "switched on" in liver cells are completely different to those that at same position in brain cells [44].

Numerous cases are born with a defect in particular gene which related to a specific illness, and this does not mean you are more susceptible to it. At the same time, this raises the risk of appearing of the disease. So, the predisposition genetic effects such as occurrence of many types of cancer may be need to be triggered by environmental factors, and to reducing the risk achieved through decreasing or avoiding such triggers [45, 46].

In each gene, non-coding regions (introns) account more than 98% and as suggested previously, they do not have any function "junk," and do not involve any information of gene output in cells. The previous opinion about non-coding DNA regions is rejected despite that role is still unknown and appears to have very important roles to do in through gene expression and regulation in each cell [47].

2.8 Genes, mutation, and single nucleotide polymorphism

As mentioned previously, about 23,000 genes in the human cell act as leader in growth and general health, which are responsible for everything in human life; in which the genetic code is a set of rules used by human being and every living system to translate the information encoded within DNA or RNA sequence to protein. Every three nucleotides called codon encode a certain amino acid in protein [48].

In this direction, any changes in the genetic code can lead to each person is exceptional in his behavior and health, that is to say, the alteration in the sequences of nucleotide in DNA can give a uniqueness characteristic for person. Mainly these changes are risk free, while others may have embroiled in proteins production either not properly, wrong sequence, or not produced totally [49]. Hence, the changes in genetic material cause inactive or disturbed gene called mutation. These mutations occur in DNA sequence either by mistake during copy process or by environmental effectors. Sometimes mutations affect individuals directly or indirectly and are prone more susceptible to certain disease circumstances [50].

3. Polymorphism

A brief glance across a time: the beginning of the human genetic polymorphism was belonging to the b globin gene in 1978, which utilized to recognize a heredity disease. After 2 years, in 1980, short distinctions in DNA discovered were spread over the whole human genome. It was described by utilized restriction fragment length polymorphisms (RFLPs) method. Further complicated interesting information of DNA polymorphisms was reported in 1985. They were named minisatellites. The empirical arguments about DNA fingerprinting remained to the 1990s. With the trial of OJ Simpson in the USA in 1995, the DNA proofs play a very important role in forensic medicine history presented by the prosecution; OJ Simpson was acquitted. This event call attention to the proofs of DNA has great significance [51].

When we see the great diversity of human ethnicities, really we find it shocking that all of these different ethnicities share a genetically identical sequence at 99%. The range of their variances is only within limits 0.1% of sequence genetic that differs between double chromosomal threads, **Figure 4**, [52, 53]. It is a small ratio of variances (1%) indeed, but it is accountable for the multiplicity in person's phenotypes and receptiveness of them to ecological contacts [53, 54].

Polymorphism at the DNA grade contains a broad domain of variations from single base pair alteration, numerous unite pairs, and frequent sequences [55]. One of the most famous types of genetic variations is the genetic mutation. Genetic mutation can be definite as order variants which happen in a smaller than 1% of the populace, whereas the extra prevalent variants are identified as polymorphisms. The greatest public hereditary variants than 1% are single nucleotide polymorphisms (SNPs) [53, 54].

Generally, genetic polymorphism can be available in numerous designs, comprising: single nucleotide polymorphisms (SNPs), tandem repeat polymorphisms which include a variable number of tandem repeats (VNTRs) and short tandem

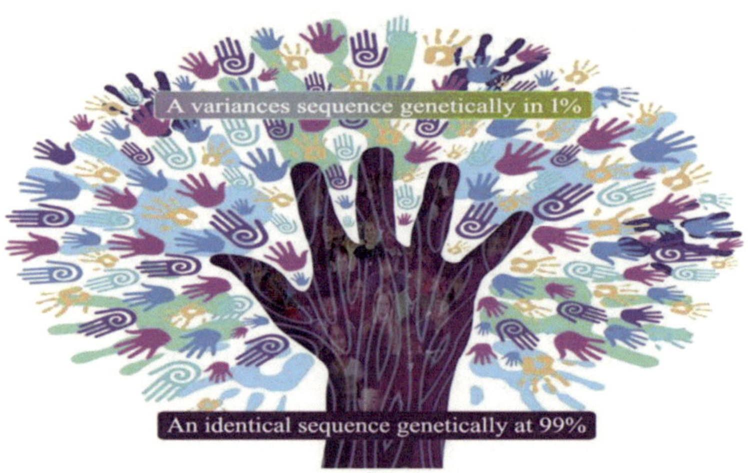

Figure 4.
Human genetic polymorphism is identical in sequences at 99% and variation sequences only about 1% [52].

repeats (STRs), insertion/deletion polymorphisms, transposable elements (TE) or Alu repeats also known as "jumping genes," structural alterations, and copy number variations (CNV) [55].

For the studying diverse kinds of DNA polymorphisms, different techniques can be utilized, such as restriction fragment length polymorphisms (RFLPs) accompanied by southern blots, polymerase chain reactions (PCRs), hybridization methods (southern and northern blotting) utilizing DNA microarray chips, and whole genome sequencing (WGS) [55]. The following is an illustration of the most famous polymorphism (**Figure 5**).

3.1 Single-nucleotide polymorphism (SNP)

Single nucleotide polymorphisms (SNPs) (pronounced: snip) are an alteration in a lone DNA order structure building block unit: (A, T, C, or G) which termed a nucleotide, **Figure 2** [56]. It is the simplest formula of genetic difference among persons. SNPs are the most frequent occurrence from all genetic variants, which happen usually in a person's DNA. It is a ratio of occurrence near 90% of human genomic variants [57, 58].

They may be occurring one time in each 300 nucleotides on usual, that is, average is about 10 million SNPs in the individual's genome. Greatest frequently, those SNPs are set between genes or within genes. They may perform as living signs and/or hereditary indicators, aiding experts find sequence, which are linked with disease. As soon as SNPs happen inside a gene or in an adjusting area nearby a gene, they might show an additional strong impact in disease via stirring the gene's role. However, the SNPs generally have no influence on the general state of health. Moreover, investigators have instituted that SNPs might assist and guess a person's reaction to definite medications. Additionally, they are utilized for a pathway of genetic factors of malady inside relatives [59–62].

3.2 Polymorphic repetitive sequences

The extension of the human genome threads that include gene sequences or intergenic and include retro (pseudo) genes and transposons are composed of small sequences of nitrogen bases that have repeated in tandem. It can consist of more two-thirds of human DNA. The number of units of these tandems in a specified site is extremely variable between separated persons. Tandem repeat polymorphisms include a variable number of tandem repeats (VNTRs) minisatellites and short tandem repeats (STRs) microsatellites. Both of VNTRs and STRs are the same in the total grounds. The difference between different alleles is consequence to a difference in the number of repeat bases that exist in alleles that are of various lengths, and later, tandem repeat polymorphisms have been identified as length polymorphisms. So, widely distinguished types from mini- and microsatellites

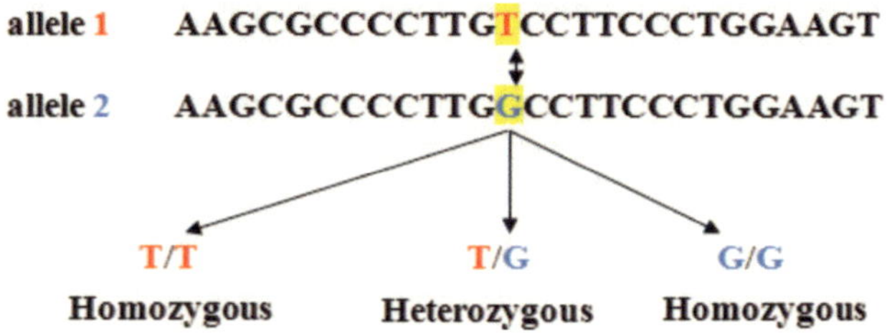

Figure 5.
Single nucleotide polymorphism for two alleles.

depend on the distance of the repeated blocks. In microsatellites, the order repeat base composes between 2 and 9 units; while mini-satellites composes between 9 and 100 units [63–65].

3.2.1 Variable number of tandem repeats (VNTRs)

VNTR is among the earliest DND markers in the application. It is a kind of tandem repetitions in which a small order of bases (10–60 base pairs) are frequented changeable times in a certain position. Therefore, VNTR is additionally familiar as minisatellites. Minisatellites are scattered everywhere in the humane DNA. Usually, the number of repeated bases in minisatellites differs among persons. Hence, the array extension shaped by VNTRs as well differs among persons. Accordingly, the variant number of chromosomes is familial from parents, so they can be applied in parental or individual identification. The techniques that use to determine this type are: routines PCR, gel electrophoresis, and amplicons of band designs by southern blotting. The utilization of VNTRs was, nevertheless, restricted by the kind of specimen that could give good results for the reason that a big quantity of DNA was needed. In addition, understanding VNTR profiles might be a difficulty. Their utilization in forensic genomics has been replaced at the present time by short tandem repeats (STRs) [66].

3.2.2 Short tandem repeats (STRs)

Short tandem repeats (STRs) give an extremely good method because of their great grade of polymorphism and a comparatively small length. Additionally, STRs are typical methods for genotyping in the identity of one's parents check and forensic identity check. A category of tandem repeats depended on presents a small order of bases (2–6 base pairs) are frequented a variable number of times in a certain site. STRs are a type of microsatellites, and they are furthermore recognized as short sequence repeats (SSRs) in plant DNA. The repeating bases consist of a single nucleotide that is familiar as a single nucleotide polymorphism (SNP) [66].

3.3 Insertion/deletion polymorphisms

It is a type of genomic difference in which a particular base order of different sizes ranging from one base to several 100 units is inserted or deleted. Indels are very extending across the DNA. Several writers consider one base pair as SNPs or frequent insertion/deletion as indels [55].

4. Genome-wide association studies (GWAS)

Genome-wide association studies (GWAS) are a new technique used worldwide in genetics research to identify inherited genetic risk variants linked with risk of prevalent disease. GWAS are the most inclusive way of genetic variation study. In general, this approach deals with full scan of genome for identifying genetic markers frequently are polymorphisms (SNPs) that appear more in patients relative to healthy individuals, and also understanding the contribution of genes in the diseases and developing better prevention and treatment approaches.

GWAS are the greatest complete way of research and contain skimming the whole genome of research members for polymorphisms and anomalies related with the sickness of attention. GWAS have the benefit of supplying a complete investigation of related genetical anomalies inside the genome, as the term "genome-wide"

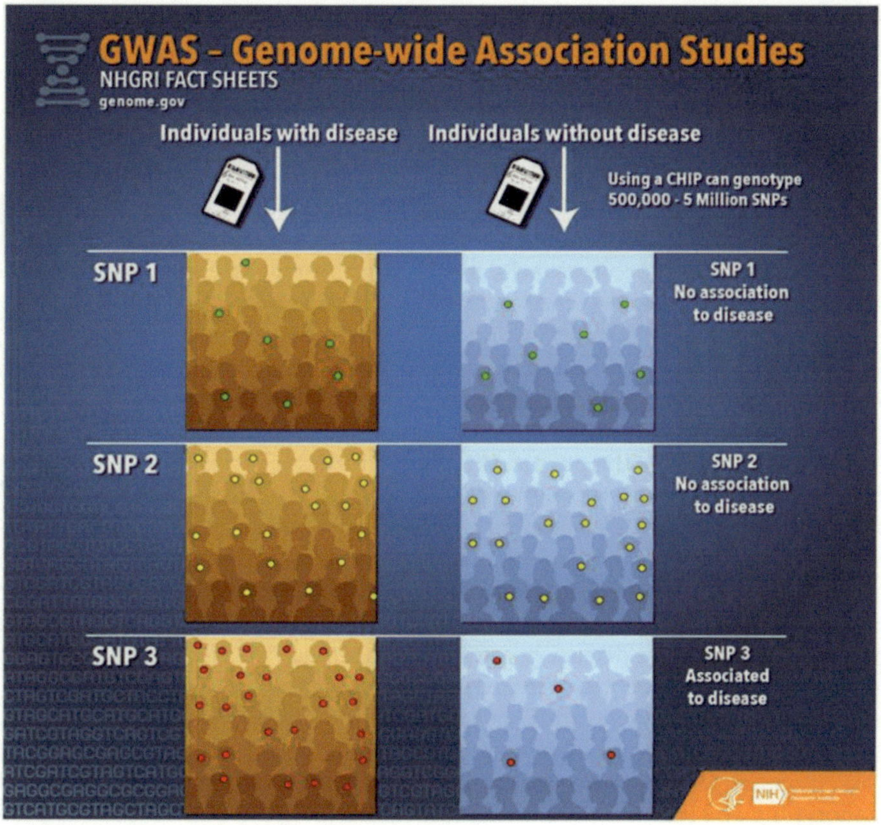

Figure 6.
Genome-wide association studies [71].

shows, in spite of that, GWAS are timing spender, costly, and yields a massive quantity of data that can/cannot actually be related to the illness of study. As of that, they are best beneficial as an initial mark pretty than a way for measuring accurate connotation [67]. In additional, GWAS are case-control study setup concentrating on obviously distinct participators geneticists who assume to find only proportionally brief extends of participate chromosomes **Figure 6** [67]. It includes comparison between two groups of individuals, one healthy and second patients or affected group with disease. Therefore, GWAS purpose is to recognize hereditary variations that convert danger of public maladies or touch additional phenotypes. The simple thought of it is: check hereditary variations (frequently SNPs), and phenotypes in haphazardly-tested persons, and view which SNPs are connected with phenotypes, while infrequent variations are inferiorly taken by GWAS method [68–70].

5. Discussion

All humans have variation in genetic material, even identical twins by the time of born, and this variation give us the uniqueness. We inherit our genes from our parents, so the members of the same family share majority of their genetic material involving its variations. The variation in DNA that cause wrong in required genetic code translates into a specific protein called pathogenic variant or mutation when linked to phenotypic particularly if they occur within the protein coding sequence of the gene. Variations are caused by the environment and genetic factors. Several disorders arise from multiple effectors like environmental, lifestyle, and genetic factors. From these diseases is behavioral genetics neuropsychiatric, such as schizophrenia, depression in which a genetic fault transferred from parents to sons through familial genes causing elevated the risk of a particular disease. SNPs can affect more than 90% of genetic variation and are responsible for the occurrence of differences between the humans. Despite the presence of SNPs, there is no relation to modify or change cellular function that is to say have no effects, and at the same time, many SNPs were found to participate in the initiation of disease like cancer or act as prophylaxis against a certain disease or even impact the responses to medications. Depending on the SNPs' position in the genome, we can classify them into that happen with exome (coding region), intron (non-coding region), and between adjacent genes (intergenic region). Because there is much of non-coding DNA (99%) that lead to harboring majority of SNPs occurring in these segments. However, only small part (1%) of genome is considered important to represent exome that can contribute existing mutations, and SNPs that have a big outcome on several diseases. Non-coding genome includes many categories of regulatory factors such as promoters, enhancers, silencers, and insulators. Each one of them provides binding sites for proteins, carries out transcription, activates transcription, suppresses transcription, and controls transcription process, respectively.

SNPs are very important and used in various studies such as estimating the tendency to disease and predicting genetic lesion; and are also used as biomarkers since they can occur near disease genes for complicated diseases, but not always. In complex disease, which means a pathological circumstance of the body due to a defect in a number of genetic and environmental aspect, SNP can affect that person has toward a specific disease. Nowadays, various methods have been established and assembled to identify known or unknown SNPs through two categories which are genotyping and scanning sequence, respectively.

Acknowledgements

I am grateful to my family, father, mother, sisters, and brothers, for always being the person I could turn to during those dark and desperate years. They sustained me in ways that I never knew that I needed.

I have to start by thanking my wife, and my daughter awesome, from reading early drafts to giving me the support. Thank you so much. "Thanks to everyone in my publishing team."

Conflict of interest

We would like to declare there is no conflict for this work.

Author details

Dhafer A.F. Al-Koofee* and Shaden M.H. Mubarak
University of Kufa, An Najaf, Iraq

*Address all correspondence to: dhafera.faisal@uokufa.edu.iq

References

[1] Ekure IA. Genetic epistemology: An examination. J. Intergative Humanism. 2015;**6**(1)

[2] Liang P, Xu Y, Zhang X, Ding C, Huang R, Zhang Z, et al. Research article Crispr/Cas9-mediated gene editing in human tripronuclear zygotes. Protein & Cell. 2015;**6**(5):363-372

[3] Chakravarti A. Perspectives on human variation through the lens of diversity and race. Cold Spring Harbor Perspectives in Biology. 2015;**7, a023358**:1-14

[4] Griffiths E, Anthony JF, Miller JH, Suzuki DT, Lewontin RC, Gelbart. Human genetics. In: An Introduction to Genetic Analysis. 7th ed. 2000

[5] Zhang W. Genetics: Analysis of genes and genomes, sixth edition. Neuro-Oncology. 2005;**7**(2):204-205

[6] Fraga Sandra Rodríguez-Rodero MF, Fernández-Morera JL, Menéndez-Torre E, Calvanese V, Fernández AF. Aging genetics and aging. Aging and Disease. 2011;**2**(3):186-195

[7] Prescott KR, Wilkie AOM. Genetics aspects of birth defects: New understandings of old problems. Archives of Disease in Childhood. Fetal and Neonatal Edition. 2007;**92**:308-314

[8] J. K. J. G. T. A. G. R. M. T. M. M. D. L. R. A. Cardiac anesthesia. Journal of Cardiothoracic and Vascular Anesthesia. 2017

[9] Zhang X, He ÃP, Liang ÃY, Yang S, Yuan ÃW, Xu S. A gene for freckles maps to chromosome 4q32–q34. The Journal of Investigative Dermatology. 2004;**122**(2):286-290

[10] Jackson M, Marks L, May GHW, Wilson JB. The genetic basis of disease. Essays in Biochemistry. 2018;**62**(December):643-723

[11] Van Loo KMJ, Martens GJM. Genetic and environmental factors in complex neurodevelopmental disorders. Current Genomics. 2007;**8**:429-444

[12] R Assessment. 3. Risk assessment. Safety Engineering. **19**:13-21

[13] Crous-Bou M, Harrington LB, Kabrhel C. Environmental and genetic risk factors associated with venous thromboembolism. Thieme E-Journals-Seminars in Thrombosis and Hemostasis. 2017;**42**(8):808-820

[14] Singh M, Tyagi SC. Ocular disorders. Genes and genetics in eye diseases: A genomic medicine approach for investigating hereditary and inflammatory ocular disorders. International Journal of Ophthalmology. 2018;**11**(1):117-134

[15] Melaiu O, Gemignani F, Landi S. The genetic susceptibility in the development of malignant pleural mesothelioma. Cancer Chemotherapy and Pharmacology. 2018;**10**(Suppl. 2): 246-252

[16] Maccoby EE. Parenting and its effects on children: On reading and misreading behavior genetics. Annual Review of Psychology. 2000;**51**:1-27

[17] Manuscript A. Overview of the genetics of major depressive disorder. Current Psychiatry Reports. 2011;**12**(6):539-546

[18] Lesch KP. CRSN symposium : Focus on depression, Part I [Symposium du CRSN : le point sur la dépression , première partie]. Gene – Environment Interaction. 2004;**29**(3):174-184

[19] Baker BJR. The cell-theory: A restatement, history, and critique

part V. The Multiplication of Nuclei. 1955;**96**:449-481

[20] Pederson T. The nucleolus. Molecular Biology of the Cell. 2011;**3**:1-15

[21] Alberts B, Johnson A, Lewis J, Raff M, Roberts K, Walter P. Copyright © 1983, 1989, 1994. Alberts B, Bray D, Lewis J, Raff M, Roberts K, Watson JD. Copyright © 2002

[22] O'Connor C, Miko I. Developing the chromosome theory. Nature Education. 2008;**1**(1):44

[23] Molecular Biology of the Cell. 2002

[24] Chueh AC, Wong LH, Wong N, Choo KHA. Variable and hierarchical size distribution of L1-retroelement-enriched CENP-A clusters within a functional human neocentromere. 2005;**14**(1):85-93

[25] Receptor E, Liehr T, Imbalances PC. Learn More about Human Chromosome Human Chromosomes Hematological Cancers. 2001

[26] Encyclopedia and Dictionary of Medicine

[27] Structural Organization of DNA

[28] Majuri I, Rautanen A. 582319 Molecular Genetics and Gene Mapping for Methodological Sciences 3 CP Course Assistants. Organizers

[29] Molecular Biology of the Cell, 4th ed

[30] Cleary MA. Autosome Learn More about Autosome Autosomes Chromosomes in the Cell. 2001

[31] Ross MT, Grafham DV, Coffey AJ, Scherer S, Mclay K, Muzny D, et al., Europe PMC Funders Group. The DNA sequence of the human X chromosome. 2009;**434**(7031):325-337

[32] Jürgen B. The fragment gene. Annals of the New York Academy of Sciences. 2009;**1178**:186-193

[33] Jo B, Choi S. Introns: The functional benefits of introns in genomes. Genomics & Informatics. 2015;**13**(4):112-118

[34] Human Genome Project Information Site Has Been Updated. Ornl.gov. 23 July 2013. Retrieved: 6 February 2014

[35] Just as reading the words on the page of a book allows an understanding of the author's message. 2016;**June**:1-5

[36] Human Genome Project Information. Genomic Science Program

[37] Allele meaning in the Cambridge English Dictionary. Dictionary.cambridge.org. [Retrieved: 29 October 2017]

[38] Genes. (n.d.). [Retrieved from: http://www.genomenewsnetwork.org/resources/whats_a_genome/Chp1_3_1.shtml#genedet8]

[39] Genetic testing. (n.d.). [Retrieved from: https://www.caregiver.org/genetic-testing]

[40] Ben-Shahar Y, Robichon A, Sokolowski M, Robinson G. Influence of gene action across different time scales on behavior. Science. 2002;**296**(5568):741-744

[41] Jirtle RL, Weidman JR. Imprinted and more equal. American Scientist. 2007;**95**:143-149

[42] Conley D, Rauscher E, Siegal ML. Beyond orchids and dandelions: Testing the 5-HTT 'risky' allele for evidence of phenotypic capacitance and frequency-dependent selection. Biodemography and Social Biology. 2013;**59**(1):37-56

[43] Takumi Takizawa TM, Meaburn KJ. The meaning of gene positioning. Cell. 2012;**135**(1):9-13

[44] Different genes are active in different kinds of cells

[45] Findlay GM, Daza RM, Martin B, et al. Accurate classification of BRCA1 variants with saturation genome editing. Nature. 2018;**562**(7726):217-222. [PubMed Abstract]

[46] Hampel H, Bennett RL, Buchanan A, et al. A practice guideline from the American College of Medical Genetics and Genomics and the National Society of genetic Counselors: Referral indications for cancer predisposition assessment. Genetics in Medicine. 2015

[47] Maston GA, Evans SK, Green MR. Transcriptional regulatory elements in the human genome. Annual Review of Genomics and Human Genetics. 2006;7:29-59

[48] Nirenberg M. Historical review: Deciphering the genetic code—A personal account. Trends in Biochemical Sciences. 2004;**29**(1):46-54. DOI: 10.1016/j.tibs.2003.11.009

[49] Griffiths AJF, Gelbart WM, Miller JH, et al. Modern Genetic Analysis. New York: W. H. Free; 1999

[50] Mutation learn science at scitable. Available from: www.nature.com. [Retrieved: 24 September 2018]

[51] Trent RJ. Forensic medicine and science. In: Molecular Medicine. Vol. 3. Amsterdam; Boston: Elsevier; 2005. pp. 221-236

[52] Faith and Service: 3 Simple Ways to Do Something—The Giving Net [Online]. Available: http://thegivingnet.com/faith-and-service-3-simple-ways-to-do-something/. [Accessed: 20 May 2019]

[53] Kruglyak L, Nickerson DA. Variation is the spice of life. Nature Genetics. 2001;**27**(3):234-236

[54] Stenson PD et al. The human gene mutation database: 2008 update. Genome Medicine. 2009;**1**(1):1-6

[55] Teama S. DNA polymorphisms: DNA-based molecular markers and their application in medicine. In: Genetic Diversity and Disease Susceptibility, i, Number Tourism. InTech; 2018. p. 13

[56] Mapping Your Health through SNPs: Your unique QR code | BioViva. [Online]. Available from: https://bioviva-science.com/blog/mapping-your-health-through-snps-your-unique-qr-code/ [Accessed: 21 May 2019]

[57] Palmer LJ, Cardon LR. Shaking the tree: Mapping complex disease genes with linkage disequilibrium. Lancet. 2005;**366**(9492):1223-1234

[58] Komar AA. Single Nucleotide Polymorphisms. Vol. 578. Totowa, NJ: Humana Press; 2009

[59] UN Library of Medicine; NIH. What are single nucleotide polymorphisms (SNPs)?—Genetics Home Reference. NIH; U.S. National Library of Medicine. [Online]. Available: https://ghr.nlm.nih.gov/primer/genomicresearch/snp

[60] Yousefi S et al. A SNP panel for identification of DNA and RNA specimens. BMC Genomics. 2018;**19**(1):1-12

[61] Huang E et al. Genome-wide screen for universal individual identification SNPs based on the HapMap and 1000 genomes databases. Scientific Reports. 2018;**8**(1):1-6

[62] Balding DJ, Martin Bishop CC. Handbook of Statistical Genetics. 3rd ed. Vol. 1. Chichester, England; Hoboken, NJ: John Wiley & Sons; 2007 Retrieved from https://www.cambridge.org/core/product/identifier/CBO9781107415324A009/type/book_part

[63] The Science of Forensic Genetics [Online]. Available from: http://www.

councilforresponsiblegenetics.org/geneticprivacy/DNA_forensics_1.html [Accessed: 23 May 2019]

[64] The Science of Forensic Genetics

[65] Panneerchelvam S, Norazmi MN. Forensic DNA profiling and database. Malaysian Journal of Medical Sciences. 2003;**10**(2):20-26

[66] Schichman SA, Suess P, Vertino AM, Gray PS. Comparison of short tandem repeat and variable number tandem repeat genetic markers for quantitative determination of allogeneic bone marrow transplant engraftment. Bone Marrow Transplantation. 2002;**29**(3):243-248

[67] Rosenfield RL, Ehrmann DA. The pathogenesis of polycystic ovary syndrome (PCOS): The hypothesis of PCOS as functional ovarian hyperandrogenism revisited. Endocrine Reviews. 2016;**37**(5):467-520. DOI: 10.1210/er.2015-1104

[68] Schwartz AG. Genetic epidemiology of cigarette smoke–induced lung disease. Proceedings of the American Thoracic Society. 2012;**9**(2):22-26

[69] Dai J. Clinical and Genetic Associations Between Lung Cancer and Chronic Obstructive Pulmonary Disease. University of Sheffield; 2017

[70] Stephens M. Statistical Genetics. 2012

[71] Genome-Wide Association Studies Fact Sheet | NHGRI. [Online]. Available from: https://www.genome.gov/about-genomics/fact-sheets/Genome-Wide-Association-Studies-Fact-Sheet [Accessed: 21 May 2019]

Chapter 2

Aldosterone Synthase Gene (*CYP11B2*) Polymorphisms and Enhanced Cardiovascular Risk

Muhammad Tarek Abdel Ghafar

Abstract

Aldosterone, the principal human mineralocorticoid, acts mainly for sodium reabsorption with potassium and hydrogen excretion. The adrenal cortex is the main site of aldosterone synthesis; however, extra-adrenal tissues such as the nervous, the cardiovascular, and the adipose tissues may be involved. Therefore, its action is mediated via endocrine as well as paracrine or autocrine mode. Aldosterone receptors are distributed extensively in the renal distal nephron and other sites, such as the heart, brain, vessels, and liver. The aldosterone synthase catalyzes the conversion of deoxycorticosterone finally to aldosterone. *CYP11B2* gene occupies human chromosome 8q21-22 with nine exons and eight introns. Alteration of aldosterone synthase gene that is attributable to genetic polymorphisms can affect its transcription leading to several cardiovascular disorders such as essential hypertension, myocardial infarction, cardiomyopathies, and atrial fibrillations. Accordingly, it is important to illustrate these polymorphisms and the mechanisms by which they alter the aldosterone synthase gene and produce cardiovascular dysfunctions.

Keywords: aldosterone, *CYP11B2*, polymorphisms, risk, transcription

1. Introduction

CYP11B2 enzyme is one of the enzymes in the pathway of steroidogenesis and responsible for the catalysis of the last three steps in the aldosterone biosynthetic cascade. It is encoded by *CYP11B2* gene located on human chromosome 8q21-22. The genetic element of cardiovascular disorders has been emerged as a risk factor for the progression of these disorders. Among these genetic elements, *CYP11B2* genetic variants and haplotypes play a pivotal role in the susceptibility, progression, survival, and therapeutic response of many cardiovascular disorders such as hypertension, coronary heart disease (CAD), atrial fibrillation (AF), cardiomyopathy, heart failure (HF), and other disorders. It was suggested to influence the cardiovascular system via alteration of aldosterone production, which acts either directly on the heart or systemically via stimulating sodium and water reabsorption and increasing the blood pressure.

2. Aldosterone

2.1 Aldosterone biosynthesis

Aldosterone is the main human mineralocorticoid. The main site of aldosterone synthesis is the zona glomerulosa (ZG) in the adrenal cortex. However, it can be produced by extra-adrenal tissues such as the central nervous system, the cardiovascular system, and the adipose tissue with a non-detectable physiological relevance and a small contribution to circulating aldosterone levels [1].

It is synthesized from cholesterol by a group of enzymatic cascade (**Figure 1**). First, cholesterol is translocated into the mitochondria across its wall mediated by steroidogenic acute regulatory protein (StAR). Cholesterol is then converted to pregnenolone, through three reactions, a 20α-hydroxylation, a 22-hydroxylation, and cleavage of the bond between C-20 and C-22 catalyzed by the *CYP11A1* cleavage enzyme, encoded by the *CYP11A1* gene on human chromosome 15 [2].

The produced pregnenolone is then released into the cytoplasm where it undergoes dehydrogenation of the 3β-hydroxyl group and isomerization of the double bond at C-5 to Δ4 by 3β-hydroxysteroid dehydrogenase (3β-HSD) and converted to progesterone [3]. Furthermore, progesterone undergoes 21-hydroxylation by the *CYP21A* enzyme encoded by *CYP21A* mapped to human chromosome 6p21·3 and located on the cytoplasmic surface of the smooth endoplasmic reticulum, generating 11-deoxycorticosterone (DOC). Then, DOC passes through three consecutive reactions catalyzed by aldosterone synthase enzyme, located on the inner mitochondrial membrane and encoded by the *CYP11B2* gene, 11β-hydroxylation to corticosterone, 18-hydroxylation to 18-hydroxycorticosterone, and finally 18-methyloxidation to aldosterone [4].

2.2 Mechanism of action of aldosterone

The action of aldosterone is mediated though mineralocorticoid receptor (MR), a specific nuclear receptor that comprises N-terminal domain, DNA-binding domain, and C-terminal ligand-binding domain. It is present as a hetero-oligomeric

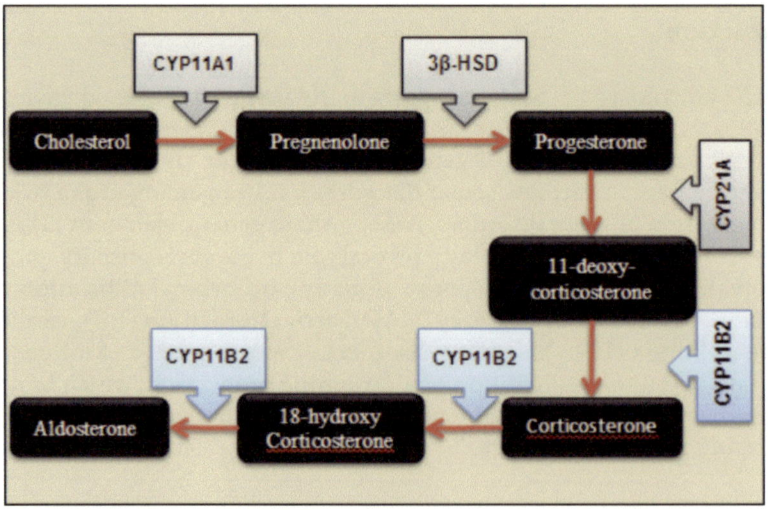

Figure 1.
Enzymatic cascade of the aldosterone biosynthesis.

complex with heat-shock proteins in the cell. Once aldosterone binds to its receptor, it undergoes a conformational change resulting in dissociation of the associated proteins, dimerization, and nuclear translocation [5]. This hormone receptor complex combines with the steroid responsive elements in the 5′-UTR of aldosterone-responsive genes with the release of aldosterone-induced proteins (AIP) that enhances or suppresses gene transcription [4].

The serine threonine glucocorticoid regulated kinase 1 (sgk1), which is one of the AIP proteins, has been phosphorylated and activated by the aldosterone, which in turn phosphorylates epithelial sodium channel (ENaC) regulatory protein, known as Nedd4–2, reducing its binding to ENaC [6] with subsequent increase in ENaC density and stability at the apical membrane resulting in increased ENaC-dependent Na^+ reabsorption [7]. The glucocorticoid-induced leucine zipper (GILZ) and the corticosteroid hormone-induced factor (CHIF) are also AIP proteins. GILZ interacts with aldosterone inhibiting the ERK signaling pathway, thus liberating ENaC from Nedd4 proteins; accordingly, its action in blocking sodium reabsorption is inhibited [8]. CHIF may affect the baso-lateral Na/K-pump, resulting in increased sodium reabsorption with potassium or hydrogen ion excretion (**Figure 2**) [9]. Aldosterone also exerts a genomic action via modulating the gene expression and subsequent protein production that result in a lag time of 1–2 h before a noticeable change in target cell activity occur [10].

2.3 Physiological action of aldosterone

As the kidneys are the main site of action for aldosterone, MRs are confined mainly in high concentration to the renal distal convoluted tubules and collecting duct controlling the apically located epithelial sodium channels at their luminal cells. Mineralocorticoid receptors also exist in other epithelial sites, such as the colon, sweat gland ducts, salivary glands [11], and non-epithelial sites including

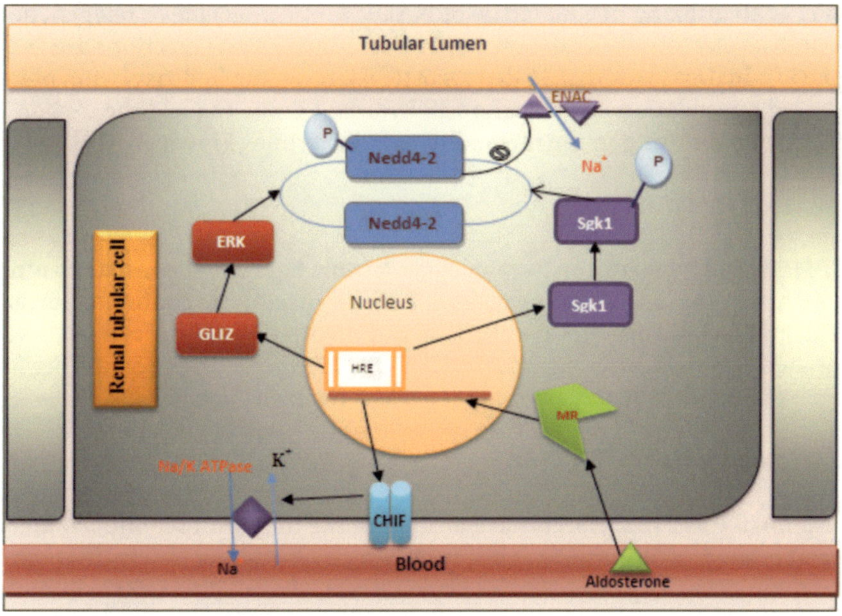

Figure 2.
Mechanism of action of aldosterone in epithelial cells. Abbreviations: ENaC, epithelial sodium channel; HRE, hormone response element; GILZ, glucocorticoid-induced leucine zipper protein; Nedd4-2, neuronal precursor cell-expressed, developmentally down-regulated protein; Sgk1, serine threonine glucocorticoid regulated kinase 1; CHIF, channel-inducing factor; MR, mineralocorticoid receptor.

myocytes, endocardium of the heart, brain, vascular smooth muscle, liver, and leukocytes [12]. The main action of aldosterone is stimulation of sodium reabsorption in the kidney and at other secretory epithelial sites with excretion of potassium and hydrogen ions [13] possibly mediated via increasing the opening periods of the existing ion channels or increasing their number [14].

In cardiovascular system, aldosterone promotes myocardial hypertrophy and fibrosis via increasing collagen I synthesis in cardiac fibroblasts and also elevating endothelin receptor numbers that further increases collagen synthesis [15]. So, increased expression of mineralocorticoid receptors in the heart may result in left-ventricular hypertrophy in normotensive subjects [16]. Aldosterone also stimulates vascular constriction via enhancing the pressor response to catecholamines and impairing the vasodilatory response to acetylcholine or by upregulation of angiotensin II receptors [4]. Also, aldosterone excess can trigger collagen deposition in blood vessels, enhancing vascular remodeling and reducing compliance [17]. In the CNS, it appears to regulate blood pressure, salt appetite, and sympathetic tone [4].

Under normal circumstances, it is likely that cardiac MRs are occupied by glucocorticoid due to its higher circulating concentration exerting antagonistic effect attenuating the rise in blood pressure and the cardiac fibrosis caused by aldosterone alone [18].

3. Cytochrome P450 11B2 (*CYP11B2*)

3.1 Reaction catalyzed

CYP11B2 enzyme is located in the inner mitochondrial membrane. Aldosterone synthesis from 11-deoxycorticosterone is catalyzed by *CYP11B2* enzyme, more commonly referred to as aldosterone synthase, which catalyzes three sequential reactions, each utilizing one molecule of NADPH, one molecule of oxygen, and the mitochondrial electron transfer system. The three sequential reactions are as follows: the 11β-hydroxylation of 11 deoxycorticosterone, the hydroxylation of carbon 18, followed by oxidation of the carbon 18 hydroxyl group to yield the carbon 18 aldehyde group resulting in the formation of aldosterone (**Figure 3**) [19].

3.2 Molecular structure

CYP11B2 gene is located on human chromosome 8q21-22. It consists of nine exons, eight introns, and comprises about 7 kb (**Figure 4**). Its coding region is 95% identical, and its intronic region is 90% identical with *CYP11B1*. However, its 5′ untranslated region is different from that of *CYP11B1* gene, thus accounting for the differences in regulation and expression pattern for each gene [20].

3.3 Protein structure

The human *CYP11B2* proteins are located in the inner mitochondrial membrane and consist of 503 amino acids, including a 24-residue N-terminal mitochondrial targeting sequence. At the protein level, the enzyme is 93% homologous with *CYP11B1* reflecting its shared 11β-hydroxylase and 18-hydroxylation activity. Only 37 amino acids differ between them which accounts for their different functions. Although *CYP11B1* and *B2* consist of the same number of amino acid, the apparent molecular mass of the human enzymes was reported as 51 and 49 kDa, respectively [20].

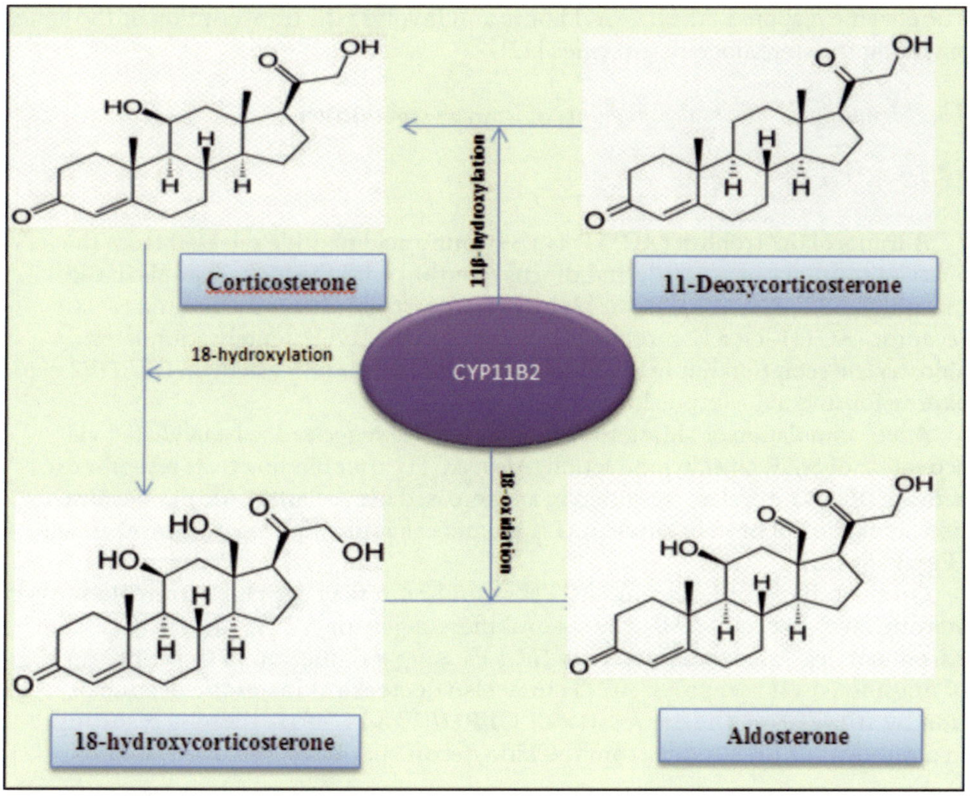

Figure 3.
Enzymatic reactions catalyzed by CYP11B2 enzyme.

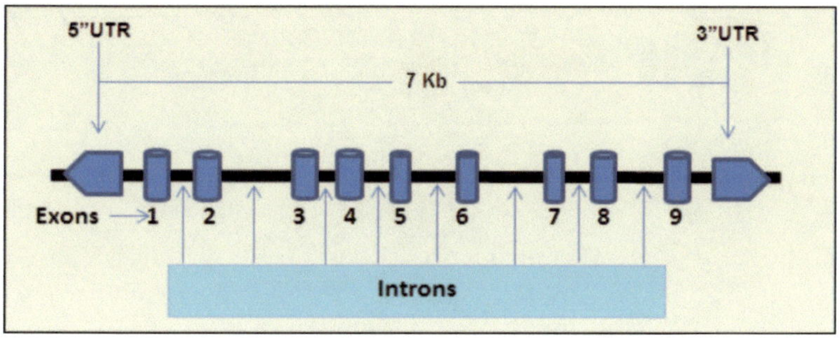

Figure 4.
Schematic diagram of the exonic-intronic arrangement of the CYP11B2 genes.

3.4 Tissue-specific expression

Expression of *CYP11B2* is limited to the adrenal cortex and appears to be exclusively in adrenal zona glomerulosa cells [21].

3.5 Regulation of *CYP11B2* expression

Adrenal steroidogenesis is under both acute and chronic regulation by tropic hormones. The acute response occurs within minutes and involves the mobilization of cholesterol from intracellular stores to the mitochondrial membrane in response to ACTH, angiotensin II, K^+, and their respective intracellular messenger pathways.

The chronic response takes several hours and involves the transcription of the genes encoding the steroidogenic enzymes [22].

3.5.1 Signaling pathways that regulate aldosterone production

3.5.1.1 ACTH

Adrenocorticotrophin (ACTH) is a 39 amino acid peptide released from the anterior pituitary in pulsatile and diurnal rhythm with the highest levels in the morning and the lowest at night [23]. ACTH exerts its effects by binding to its receptor (ACTH-R), a G-protein-coupled receptor. ACTH acutely stimulates aldosterone secretion but in the long term has an inhibitory effect on *CYP11B2* gene expression and aldosterone levels [24].

Acute stimulation of aldosterone production has suggested to be mediated via activation of StAR protein production. Also, ACTH after binding to its receptor can activate adenylate cyclase, resulting in an increased intracellular cAMP concentration, activation of protein kinase A (PKA), and calcium influx via calcium channels (**Figure 5**) [25].

On the other hand, chronic ACTH stimulation may depress serum aldosterone level as cyclic AMP, the second messenger for ACTH, desensitizes adrenocortical cells to angiotensin II by causing a reduction in the expression of angiotensin II receptors. ACTH may also decrease aldosterone production by stimulating the expression of *CYP11B1* and *CYP17*, thereby resulting in a removal of precursors from the aldosterone pathway and using them to

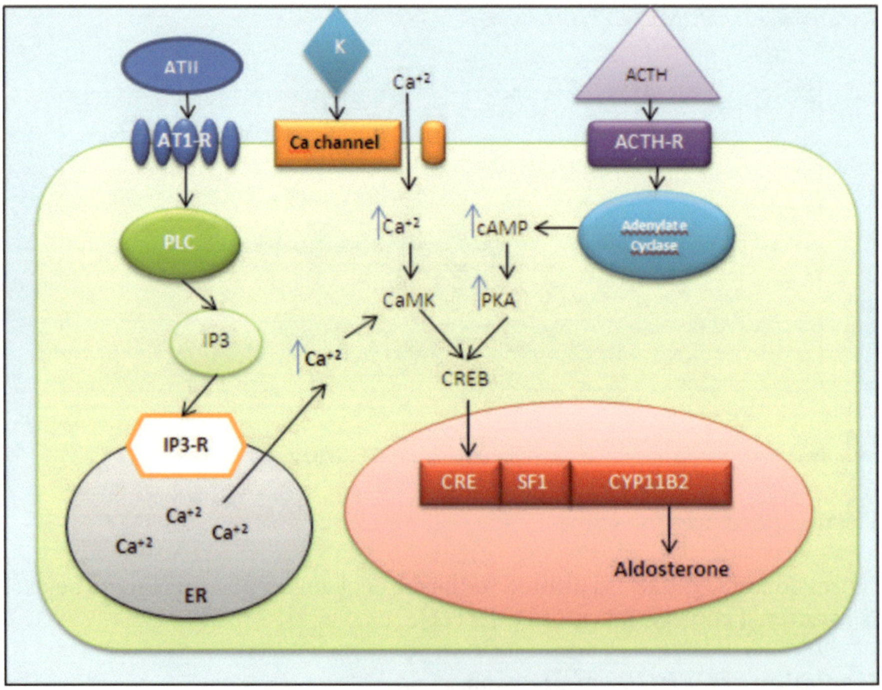

Figure 5.
Intracellular mechanisms of angiotensin II, K$^+$ *and ACTH influencing gene expression. Abbreviations: ER, endoplasmic reticulum; AT1-R, angiotensin 1 receptor; PLC, phospholipase C; PKA, protein kinase A; IP3R, inositol triphosphate receptor; IP3, inositol triphosphate; CaMK, calmodulin kinase; SF-1, steroidogenic factor 1; CREB, cAMP regulatory element response element; ACTH, adrenocorticotrophic hormone.*

synthesize cortisol. ACTH appears to specifically induce the proliferation of zona fasciculata cells while recruiting and transforming glomerulosa cells into fasciculata-like cells [26].

Under normal circulating ACTH levels, the glomerulosa maintains *CYP11B2* expression by at least two mechanisms. First, angiotensin II inhibits ACTH-stimulated cAMP production in glomerulosa but not fasciculata cells. Second, the glomerulosa expresses a type of adenyl cyclase that is inhibited by increasing intracellular Ca^{2+}, the second messenger for both angiotensin II and K^+ [27].

3.5.1.2 Angiotensin II

Angiotensin II is thought to stimulate aldosterone synthesis as result of sodium depletion and extracellular fluid volume reduction through various intracellular signaling pathways. However, the best characterized pathway is the activation of phospholipase C (**Figure 5**). It is mediated by acting on angiotensin 1 (AT1) receptor, a specific G-protein-coupled receptor that activates phospholipase C. Once activated, phospholipase C hydrolyses phosphatidyl inositol 4,5-biphosphate (PIP2) to 1,4,5 inositol triphosphate (IP3) and 1,2-diacylglycerol (DAG) resulting in release of Ca^{2+} from intracellular stores and activation of protein kinase C (PKC), respectively. The increased intracellular Ca^{2+} concentration activates calmodulin and Ca^{2+}/calmodulin-dependent protein kinases (CaM kinases) [28, 29] to phosphorylate and activate transcription factors as activating transcription factor 1 (ATF-1), cAMP-response-element binding protein (CREB), nerve growth factor IB (NGFIB), and nuclear receptor related 1 protein (*NURR1*) that combined to specific cis-acting series in the 5′ region of *CYP11B2* [30]. The acute stimulation mediated by angiotensin II can stimulate rapid aldosterone synthesis either de novo or from intermediate compounds in the steroidogenic pathway. However, chronic stimulation may lead to ZG hypertrophy and hyperplasia with increased *CYP11B2* expression and subsequent aldosterone secretion [31].

3.5.1.3 Potassium

The level of potassium affects renin secretion as well as having a direct effect on the adrenal cortex to increase aldosterone secretion. Increased extracellular K^+ (like angiotensin II) stimulates aldosterone secretion through an increase in intracellular Ca^{2+} and activation of calmodulin kinases with consequent phosphorylation of transcription factors leading to stimulation of *CYP11B2* gene transcription. Potassium signaling is mediated through membrane depolarization, leading to an influx of calcium through T and L-type channels (**Figure 5**) [32].

3.5.2 Transcriptional regulation of CYP11B2 gene

As mentioned previously, chronic regulation of steroidogenesis involves transcription of the genes encoding the necessary steroidogenic enzymes. This is mediated by alteration of trans-acting factors that bind to the cis-regulatory elements within the 5′ regulatory regions of the target genes. Investigation of the 5′ regulatory regions of the *CYP11B* gene revealed six cis-acting elements (Ad1–6) (**Figure 6**). The most important cis-elements in the *hCYP11B2* promoter are CRE at −71/−64 (Ad1), Ad5 at −129/−114, Ad4 at −344/−336, and a cis-element termed NGFIB response element 1 (NBRE-1) −766/−759 (**Figure 7**) [33].

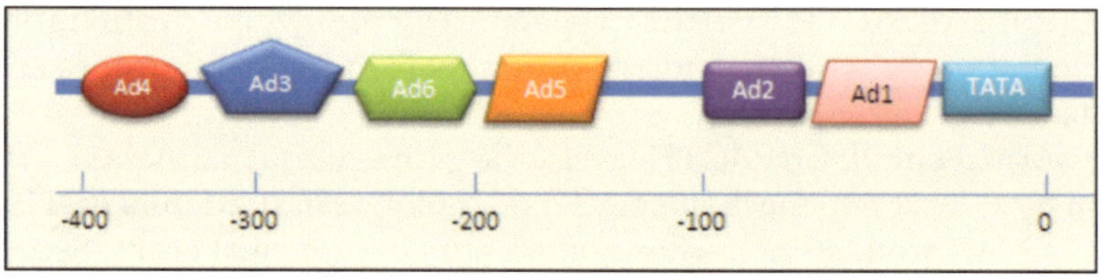

Figure 6.
Schematic diagram of the CYP11B2 promoter with the cis-elements (Ad1–Ad6).

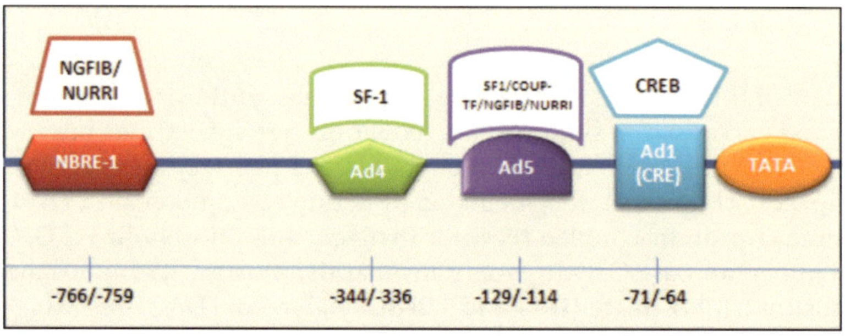

Figure 7.
Schematic diagram of the most important transcription factor binding sites in the hCYP11B2 5'UTR. Abbreviations: CREB, cAMP regulatory element response element; SF-1, steroidogenic factor 1; COUP-TF, chicken ovalbumin upstream promoter transcription factor; NGFIB, nerve growth factor IB; NURRI, nuclear receptor-related 1 protein; NBRE-1, NGFI-B response element.

3.5.2.1 Ad1 (CRE)

The Ad1 element closely resembles a consensus cAMP regulatory element (CRE) site. CREs plays an essential role in cAMP-dependent gene expression of a wide variety of genes. Proteins, such as the CRE-binding protein (CREB) and the highly related activating transcription factors (ATF), bind to CRE sites to initiate transcription. CREB binds to DNA as a dimer and has a conserved region of leucine residues (leucine zipper) at its C terminus that enables dimerization and sequence specific DNA binding [34].

CREB functions not only as a component of a variety of signaling pathways, particularly PKA, but also mitogen-activated protein kinases (MAPKs) and CaMKs. All these pathways mediate CREB-induced transcription by phosphorylating CREB at residue serine 133 [35]. The phosphorylated serine 133 binds another protein referred to as the CREB-binding protein (CBP). CBP is a 265-kDa nuclear protein, which binds to phosphorylated CREB and allows recruitment and stabilization of the RNA polymerase II transcription complex on the promoter of CREB target genes [36].

Using electrophoretic mobility shift assay, the *CYP11B2* CRE has been shown to bind members of the activating transcription factor (ATF-1 and ATF-2) and CRE-binding protein (CREB) families. The ability of these transcription factors, particularly ATF-1 and CREB, to enhance transcription is partially regulated by their state of phosphorylation. Thus, one possibility is that activated CaMK I or CaMK IV phosphorylates CREB or ATF-1 leading to increased *CYP11B2* transcription [28].

3.5.2.2 AD4 (SF-1)

The Ad4 site (CCAAGGTC) is also found to be important in the regulation of the *CYP11B* gene. This Ad4 site or homologous sequences have been identified in the regulatory regions of all other steroid P450 genes (*CYP11A1*, *CYP21*, *CYPI7*, *CYP11B1*,

CYP11B2, and *CYPI9*), suggesting an important functional role in steroidogenesis. An Ad4-binding protein (Ad4BP) has been identified and cloned from bovine adrenal cortex nuclear extract. Ad4BP is a homolog of the steroidogenic factor 1 (SF-1) identified in the human [37].

SF-1 is an orphan member of the nuclear hormone receptor superfamily, with potential phosphorylation sites for cAMP-dependent kinases, CaMK or PKC, suggesting a role for SF-1 in cAMP-dependent transcription. SF-1 is a 53 kDa protein consisting of a zinc finger domain and ligand binding/dimerization domain. The hydroxyl cholesterols enhance SF-1-dependent transcriptional activity in vitro, suggesting that SF-1 is a ligand-activated receptor. However, this is a controversial finding and needs further clarification [38].

SF-1 is expressed exclusively in steroidogenic tissues and plays an essential role in the development and function of the primary steroidogenic tissues [39]. Within the adrenal, SF-1 has been found to play a key role in the transcriptional regulation of most of the steroid hydroxylase genes (*CYP11A1*, *CYP21*, *CYP11B1*, *CYP17*, and *CYP 19*) as well as three *β HSD* and steroidogenic *acute regulatory protein* (StAR). SF-1 regulation of transcription is mediated by interaction with various co-activator proteins, including steroid receptor coactivator 1 (SRC1), glucocorticoid receptor interacting protein (GRIP), and also through repressors such as dosage-sensitive adrenal hypoplasia congenita of the X chromosome 1 (DAX1) that inhibits SF-1-mediated steroidogenesis [40].

The Ad4 or SF-1 site has been identified in all steroid P450s based on sequence alignments, including at position −351/−343 (AGGTCC) of *CYP11B2.* Although this site binds strongly to SF-1, deletion studies suggest that it is not essential for basal or stimulus-induced expression of *CYP11B2*. In fact, co-expression of *CYP11B2* reporter gene constructs with SF-1 has a negative effect on gene transcription, making the regulation of *CYP11B2* different to the other steroidogenic genes, *StAR*, *CYP11A*, *CYP11B1*, and *CYP 17* that are all induced by SF-1. The effects of both NGFIB and NURRl on *CYP11B2* expression can be inhibited by SF-1 supporting a negative effect of SF-1 [33]. Thus, *hCYP11B2* expression is regulated quite differently from genes for other proteins involved in steroid biosynthesis including *StAR*, *CYP11A*, *CYP11B1*, and *CYP17*, which are all positively regulated by SF-1 [41].

3.5.2.3 AD5

Electrophoretic mobility shift assay (EMSA) analysis of the −129/−114 (Ad5) element (CTCCAGCCTTGACCTT) has shown that it binds several nuclear proteins, including SF-1 and another orphan nuclear receptor, chicken ovalbumin upstream promoter transcription factor (COUP-TF). On the bovine *CYP 17* and the mouse *CYP21* gene, COUP-TF and SF-1 bind competitively to a common site. Deletion of this site decreases basal activity by approximately 80% and also reduces the maximal response to Ca^{2+} and cAMP stimulation [42].

3.5.2.4 NBRE

The transcription factors nerve growth factor IB (NGFIB) and nuclear receptor-related 1 protein (NURRl) are members of the NGFIB family of orphan nuclear receptors that bind to a consensus sequence NGFI-B response element (NBRE) (AAAGGTCA). These factors can also bind to the Ad5 element as well as a novel NBRE-1 site at −766/−759. Both these transcription factors increase *CYP11B2* expression by angiotensin II or K^+ stimulation. Mutation of the NBRE-1 site decreases basal expression as well as the response to angiotensin II and K^+.

Therefore, the CRE, Ad5, and NBRE-1 sites interact to regulate basal transcription as well as the response to each signaling pathway (cAMP or Ca^{2+}) [33].

4. Genotypic variants and haplotypes in *CYP11B2* gene

Several polymorphisms have been identified in *CYP11B2* and are associated with enhanced *CYP11B2* transcription, increased aldosterone production, and the progression of many cardiovascular disorders (**Figure 8**). About 227 single-nucleotide polymorphisms (SNPs) have been detected in different population worldwide according to National Center for Biotechnology Information (NCBI) database (https://www.ncbi.nlm.nih.gov/) [43]. However, only few SNPs are evaluated in different studies. The first and most extensively studied polymorphism is −344 C/T which exists in the 5′ promoter region of *CYP11B2* gene. It occupies the putative binding site for the transcription factor SF-1 which is responsible for the expression of several enzymes involved in steroid biosynthesis framework in the adrenal cortex. The two alternative bases at this position are thymine (T) and cytosine (C) [44]. *CYP11B2* −344C/T polymorphism is associated with increased aldosterone synthesis and secretion in serum [45] or urine [46] and increased aldosterone renin ratio [47, 48] with either C allele or T allele were suggested to be involved among different studies. The mechanisms that stand behind this association are conflicting. Functional studies showed that T allele binds to SF-1 with four folds lower affinity than the C allele. This results in stimulation of the expression of enzymes responsible for steroidogenesis leading to increased aldosterone synthase activity in C allele carriers [41]. However, in T allele carrier, the increased aldosterone production was explained by lower affinity for SF1 binding leading to the increased availability of this transcription factor in other parts of the gene with subsequent activation of the steroidogenic acute regulatory gene [45]. On the other hand, others suggest that this polymorphism exert its effect via a strong linkage disequilibrium with functional polymorphisms in *CYP11B1*, a substitution (T to C) in codon 75 and (G to A) in intron 6 that result in 11 β hydroxylase deficiency [49]. This results in sustained elevation of ACTH [50] with subsequent increases in the expression of a number of genes required for aldosterone synthesis including StAR, *CYP11A*, and *CYP21* leading to enhanced aldosterone synthesis [31, 50].

The second polymorphism is a gene intronic conversion (IC) whereby a fragment of the "wild-type (Wt)" intron 2 of *CYP11B2* is replaced by the corresponding intronic fragment of *CYP11B1* conversion (Conv). Due to the nature of this variation and difficulty in genotyping it, its frequency has not been reported in

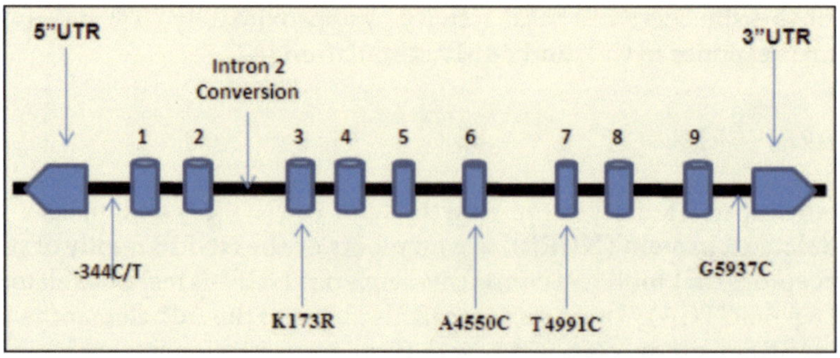

Figure 8.
Common CYP11B2 polymorphisms associated with increased aldosterone production.

public databases. The −344 T/C and intron conversion polymorphisms are in tight linkage disequilibrium and three common haplotypes have been reported: T/Conv (38%), C/Wt (45%), and T/Wt (13%), where the first allele corresponds to the −344 polymorphism (T or C) and the second to the intron 2 conversion (Wt or Conv) [31].

Beside the previously described polymorphisms of *CYP11B2*, other interesting polymorphisms have been reported and associated with increased aldosterone production as missense mutation in exon 3, where a lysine is replaced by an arginine (K173R) and *CYP11B2* (T4991C) SNP in exon 7 [51]. However, the haplotype including −344T and K173 was associated with higher *CYP11B2* expression in adrenal tissue than the −344C and R173 haplotype [52]. Moreover, other polymorphisms have been studied as G5937C and A4550C and were associated with heart size [53].

4.1 *CYP11B2* genotypic variants and hypertension

Hypertension is a complex progressive cardiovascular disorder, not just a scale of threshold blood pressure values, with many causes that result in both functional and structural cardiac and vascular system abnormalities that damage the heart, kidneys, brain, vasculature, and other organs, and lead to premature morbidity and death [54]. Essential hypertension is a multifactorial disorder, predisposed by genetic and environmental factors [55]. Growing evidences suggest the potential role of genetic alteration affecting genes encoding the aldosterone synthesis pathway enzymes with associated enhanced aldosterone production resulting in progression to essential hypertension [56].

Several polymorphic variants of *CYP11B2* have been identified as potential genetic contributor in patients with essential hypertension with −344C/T was extensively studied among different ethnic groups, with conflicting results. Public databases reported that the T allele is more frequent than the C allele in highlanders compared with lowlanders Indian [57], African Americans and Japanese subjects [48], Caucasian [58], Tamil population [59], Chinese Han population [38], Taiwanese females [60], and recently in the Egyptian population [61]. C allele has been suggested to be associated with hypertension by Tsukada et al. [62], Kumar et al. [63], Ji et al. [64], Li et al. [65], and in the meta-analysis by Cheng et al. [66]. No association was detected in the Japanese population [67] and in the meta-analysis by Chen et al. [68]. These discrepancies reflect the influence of different genetic and environmental factors as well as the age and gender in geographically separated populations [61].

The *CYP11B2* gene intronic conversion (IC) was also described in a small study of essential hypertensive subjects; the conversion allele frequency was much lower in black subjects compared with white [69]. However, several studies proved the more frequent association of *CYB11B2* −344T/IC haplotype with hypertensive subjects than normotensives, especially those with a high aldosterone renin ratio (ARR) and increased aldosterone levels in plasma [45, 47], although this finding is not supported in all studies [67]. IC has also associated with a better therapeutic response to anti-hypertensive treatment [70].

On the other hand, *CYP11B2* (K173R) and *CYP11B2* (T4991C) polymorphisms were found to be associated with hypertension [51, 52]. A strong synergistic effect has existed among different genotypes of *CYP11B2* C−344T, IC, and K173R polymorphisms with the haplotype (−344T-Conv-K173) associated with a higher risk for essential hypertension progression [43]. Despite the use of several polymorphisms in *CYP11B2,* their causal relationship with hypertension and inappropriate aldosterone production remains unclear.

4.2 *CYP11B2* genotypic variants and atrial fibrillation

Atrial fibrillation (AF) is the most clinically prevalent type of cardiac arrhythmia which may be precipitated due to the presence of underlying heart disease such as valvular dysfunction, ventricular dysfunction, and hypertension. However, AF does not exist in some patients with one or more of these risk factors and presents in others without any risk factors. Accordingly, the genetic role had been emerged in the predisposition for AF. A positive family history of AF in at least one parent was suggested by a recent Framingham Heart study on 2243 participants to be associated with an 85% increased relative risk for AF [71].

Taking together this genetic role, two types of AF have been identified regarding the heredity characteristics as familial and non-familial AF. Recent studies have detected several candidate genes which were suggested to be associated with the familial AF type such as genes encoding for subunits of potassium or sodium channels, sarcolipin, connexin 40, endothelial nitric oxide synthase, interleukin 10, and RAAS [72].

Association of genetic variants of renin angiotensin aldosterone system (RAAS) system with non-familial AF was suggested by Tsai et al. [73] using a risk-factor matched design. *CYP11B2* −344C/T polymorphism was reported to be associated with the susceptibility of AF by Amir et al. [74] in a cohort of 196 patients with symptomatic systolic heart failure. They found that the −344 CC genotype to be a strong independent predictor for AF (adjusted OR 2.35, 95% CI 1.57–3.51, $P = 0.03$). Therefore, *CYP11B2* −344C/T polymorphism may predispose to AF in patients with HF. Another study by Lu et al. [75] on 359 of Han and Kazak population with non-valvular AF and 527 non-AF patients as a control reported that −344C/T polymorphism of *CYP11B2* was associated with AF risk as the frequencies of TT genotype, and co-dominant model (CC + TT genotype) in Han population and of TT genotype, and dominant model (CT + TT genotype) in Kasak population were significantly higher in AF group than in the control group. Furthermore, a meta-analysis by Li et al. [76] involving 2758 subjects from six distinct studies reported that *CYP11B2* T−344C gene polymorphism was significantly associated with AF in all genetic models; allelic (OR: 1.26, $P = 0.0002$), recessive (OR: 1.99, $P = 0.003$), dominant (OR: 0.903, $P = 0.036$), and homozygous (OR: 1.356, 95% CI: 1.130–1.628, $P = 0.001$), and additive (OR: 1.153, $P = 1.0 \times 10^{-10}$). On the other hand, no significant association was detected by Zhang et al. [77] between different genotype and alleles of −344 T/C polymorphism and lone AF patients.

The possible mechanisms for the association of *CYP11B2* polymorphism and AF are mainly related to increased aldosterone production. Aldosterone exerts its effect via direct and indirect ways. Indirect effect of aldosterone on the heart arise from its role on increasing blood volume, blood pressure, left ventricular pressure, left ventricular hypertrophy, left atrial pressure, and left atrial volume. However, aldosterone can directly act on the heart inducing cardiac hypertrophy and fibrosis [78, 79] via the proliferation and differentiation of myocardial cells, vascular smooth muscle cells, and fibroblasts, leading to a significant increase in collagen production. These effects lead to cardiac fibrosis and structural remodeling leading to heart rhythm disorders. Specifically, in the atrium, aldosterone may directly or indirectly cause atrial enlargement and fibrosis, leading to structural and electrical atrial remodeling resulting in atrial fibrillation. Based on these findings, aldosterone antagonists as angiotensin II receptor antagonists may be used clinically in the patients with AF to control and minimize the incidence and persistence of AF [80].

4.3 *CYP11B2* genotypic variants and coronary artery disease

Coronary artery disease (CAD) is a complex disorder comprised two major subsequent events: coronary atherosclerosis and myocardial infarction (MI). Despite the major progress in diagnosis of CAD, the pathogenesis and possible risk factors need further evaluation. The classical risk factors including positive family history, smoking, high body mass index, and disorders as hyperlipidemia, hypertension, and diabetes mellitus have been reported to be responsible for no more than 50% of total risk factors for CAD. Accordingly, genetic background seems also to participate in the predisposition for CAD [81].

Among the different polymorphisms described for *CYP11B2* gene, several studies have shown that the *CYP11B2* gene -344T>C polymorphism is associated with CAD in different ethnic groups with controversial results. Previous study on 201 CAD patients and 201 controls form Italian population have detected that *CYP11B2* polymorphism and CC genotype were associated with CAD risk in crude analysis with borderline significance which is lost by stratification to the confounding factors as smoking and family history [82]. A meta-analysis suggested that the −344T>C polymorphism in the *CYP11B2* gene might be associated with susceptibility to CAD in Caucasians and Asians [83]. A study on 609 Taiwanese male and female subjects who were unrelated and received coronary catheterization found that the C/C allele occurred more frequently in females who had CAD, and that it was associated with higher left ventricular mass (LVM) and left ventricular end diastolic diameter (LVEDD) [84]. Sharma et al. [85] also reported the association of the *CYP11B2* −344C>T polymorphism with the size of atherosclerotic plaque in the carotid artery. Neal et al. [86] suggested that −344C/T polymorphism is a cardiovascular risk factor due to its association with LV hypertrophy and decreased baroreflex sensitivity which predict the morbidity and mortality rates of MI. Others failed to find any significant association of *CYP11B2* with CAD in different populations as in an Indian population and other populations [87–89].

The underlying mechanism by which the *CYP11B2* -344T>C polymorphism can increase the risk for CAD remains unclear. However, it is related to its effect on increasing expression of *CYP11B2*, thereby increasing aldosterone secretion [83]. Also, the influence of gene-environment interaction has been involved as an etiological factor for CAD risk. Growing evidence has suggested the interaction between -344T>C polymorphism and positive smoking for enhanced CAD risk [90]. Also, Hautanen et al. [91] detected that smoking and dyslipidemia are associated risk factors for non-fatal MI in males who were carriers for *CYP11B2* −344C/T allele.

4.4 *CYP11B2* genotypic variants and hypertrophic cardiomyopathy

Hypertrophic cardiomyopathy (HCM) is a clinical cardiac dysfunction characterized mainly by hypertrophy of left ventricle. HCM is an autosomal dominant disorder and its diagnosis needs to exclude other cardiac or systemic causes of increased ventricular wall thickening. HCM comprises different histological features as cardiomyocyte hypertrophy, myofibrillar disarray, and fibrosis. Several factors are involved in the pathogenesis of HCM, with the genetic element has an upper hand. Mutations and polymorphisms in genes encoding the sarcomere proteins and renin-angiotensin-aldosterone system (RAAS) seem to be related to the predisposition for left ventricular hypertrophy (LVH) and HCM [92].

Evidences suggested that aldosterone seems to play a major role in the progression of LVH and HCM as it is produced locally in the heart and *CYP11B2* mRNA levels show sevenfold increase in the cardiac tissue of HCM patients when compared normal cardiac tissue [93]. It exerts its action via stimulation of mineralocorticoid receptor resulting in enhancement of myocardial cell hypertrophy, progressive myocardial fibrosis leading to ventricular and septal remodeling, and hypertrophy, resulting in elevated ventricular mass observed in HCM patients [94, 95]. Therefore, genetic variations involving *CYP11B2* gene might influence the structure and function of the left ventricle via increasing aldosterone secretion [93].

Several polymorphisms in the *CYP11B2* had been described in the HCM with −344C>T and intron 2 conversion have significant associations with left ventricular size, mass, and function in different population studies. However, the −344C>T promoter polymorphism is a much better predictor of left ventricular size than is the intron 2 gene conversion [96]. The −344C>T polymorphism have proved to be associated with the risk for HCM progression in many previous studies [93, 94, 97–99], whereas no association has suggested by other studies [100, 101].This controversy extents to the risk allele, which may be the −344C in some studies [96, 98–100, 102, 103] or −344T in another study [97]. Moreover, the risk allele for increased ventricular size and thickness differs regarding gender as with a study by Chai et al., [97] in which the T allele carrier is associated with a significantly higher intra-ventricular septum thickness in males, whereas in females, CC genotype carriers had a higher risk for increased intra-ventricular mass thickness, left ventricular mass index, and Wigle score.

4.5 *CYP11B2* genotypic variants and heart failure

Heart failure (HF) is a cardiac disorder characterized by cardiac remodeling with subsequent cardiac dysfunction [104]. It is a multifactorial disease, which is precipitated due to underlying cardiac disorders as hypertension, CAD, valvular dysfunction, arrhythmia, and cardiomyopathy. Integrated neuronal and hormonal elements are involved in the pathogenesis of HF including activation of the sympathetic nervous system and the renin-angiotensin-aldosterone system, and other mediators as endothelin, vascular endothelial growth factor, and inflammatory cytokines. Based on the previously described neurohormonal factors, therapeutic approaches for HF have developed to block these factors including angiotensin-converting enzyme inhibitors (ACEI), and aldosterone antagonists [105]. Several risk and prognostic factors have influenced the progression of chronic congestive heart failure (CHF) including age, New York Heart Association (NYHA) class, renal function, and comorbidities such as atrial fibrillation, diabetes mellitus, and ischemic heart disease [106]. However, genetic elements seem to affect the risk, severity, and therapeutic response of HF [107]. *CYP11B2* polymorphisms specifically −344C/T is among these genetic factors and has been associated with the susceptibility, therapeutic response, or prognosis of HF.

A study by McNamara et al. [108] was performed on a total of 354 subjects from A-HeFT (African American Heart Failure Trial). They detected a higher frequency of −344 TT genotypes carriers (61%) than CC genotypes carriers (6.2%) in African Americans. Also, the −344 C allele was associated with significantly poorer HF hospitalization-free survival and a higher rate of death. Moreover, the therapeutic influence of nitric oxide donor (isosorbide dinitrate and hydralazine) was augmented in the presence of the TT genotype.

Another study by Feola et al. [109] on 175 patients from the European continental ancestry congestive heart failure (CHF) population and revealed that no significant differences between −344 CC and −344 TT genotypes carriers regarding cardiac output, end-systolic or diastolic left ventricle diameter, left ventricular ejection fraction (LVEF), and pro-natriuretic peptide (BNP). Also, −344 C allele carriers have a higher degree of disability (Barthel Index), NYHA class, and a lower cardiac index. Moreover, the two groups showed a similar clinical outcomes either death or re-hospitalization after 4 years follow up period.

In 107 Black South African patients with dilated cardiomyopathy in functional class II–III, Tiago et al. [110] detected that the −344C allele was associated with improvement of LVEF after traditional therapy despite it is not related to the baseline LVEF as well as left ventricular dimension. Also, the allele distribution has proven to be different among races as the C allele was significantly more frequent in non-African-American HF patients if compared with African-American patients and associated only in the African-American with a lower end-systolic left ventricular diameter at 1 year follow-up [111]. Moreover, the association of −344C allele was confirmed as a risk factor for the progression of AF in a cohort of 194 African-American HF patients [112].

5. Conclusions

CYP11B2 gene polymorphism is associated with increased cardiovascular risk via enhancing aldosterone synthesis and production which acts either systemically or locally on the heart. There is a large number of polymorphisms has been identified for *CYP11B2*. Among them, −344C/T polymorphism was extensively studied in different ethnic groups and has proved to be associated either solely or synergistic with other *CYP11B2* polymorphisms in the risk for progression and susceptibility of several cardiovascular disorders as hypertension, AF, CAD, cardiomyopathy, and HF. Also, *CYP11B2* polymorphisms were confirmed as a predictor for survival and therapeutic response in some cardiovascular disorders as hypertension and HF. Moreover, gene-environment interactions of *CYP11B2* were suggested in several studies but still need to be confirmed.

Thanks

First of all thanks to gracious ALLAH who guided me to the frank clear way. Second, I dedicate this work to my parents and my dear professor Murad Ahmad Murad for their encouragement and sustained support. And finally, I am grateful to my lovely niece, Marium.

Author details

Muhammad Tarek Abdel Ghafar
Clinical Pathology Department, Faculty of Medicine, Tanta University, Tanta, Egypt

*Address all correspondence to: mohammedtarek5514@yahoo.com

References

[1] Davies E, MacKenzie SM. Extra-adrenal production of corticosteroids. Clinical and Experimental Pharmacology & Physiology. 2003;**30**(7):437-445

[2] Stocco DM. StAR protein and the regulation of steroid hormone biosynthesis. Annual Review of Physiology. 2001;**63**:193-213

[3] Lieberman S, Lin YY. Reflections on sterol sidechain cleavage process catalyzed by cytochrome P450(scc). The Journal of Steroid Biochemistry and Molecular Biology. 2001;**78**(1):1-14

[4] Connell JM, Davies E. The new biology of aldosterone. The Journal of Endocrinology. 2005;**186**(1):1-20

[5] Rogerson FM, Brennan FE, Fuller PJ. Mineralocorticoid receptor binding, structure and function. Molecular and Cellular Endocrinology. 2004;**217**(1-2):203-212

[6] Naray-Fejes-Toth A, Helms MN, Stokes JB, Fejes-Toth G. Regulation of sodium transport in mammalian collecting duct cells by aldosterone-induced kinase, SGK1: Structure/function studies. Molecular and Cellular Endocrinology. 2004;**217**(1-2):197-202

[7] Snyder PM, Olson DR, Thomas BC. Serum and glucocorticoid-regulated kinase modulates Nedd4-2-mediated inhibition of the epithelial Na^+ channel. The Journal of Biological Chemistry. 2002;**277**(1):5-8

[8] Bhalla V, Soundararajan R, Pao AC, Li H, Pearce D. Disinhibitory pathways for control of sodium transport: Regulation of ENaC by SGK1 and GILZ. American Journal of Physiology. Renal Physiology. 2006;**291**(4):F714-F721

[9] Chatterjee VK, Beck-Peccoz P. Hormone-nuclear receptor interactions in health and disease: Thyroid hormone resistance. Baillière's Clinical Endocrinology and Metabolism. 1994;**8**(2):267-283

[10] Losel R, Schultz A, Wehling M. A quick glance at rapid aldosterone action. Molecular and Cellular Endocrinology. 2004;**217**(1-2):137-141

[11] Pearce D, Bhargava A, Cole TJ. Aldosterone: Its receptor, target genes, and actions. Vitamins and Hormones. 2003;**66**:29-76

[12] Gomez-Sanchez EP, Ahmad N, Romero DG, Gomez-Sanchez CE. Origin of aldosterone in the rat heart. Endocrinology. 2004;**145**(11):4796-4802

[13] Horisberger JD. Amiloride-sensitive Na channels. Current Opinion in Cell Biology. 1998;**10**(4):443-449

[14] Kim GH, Masilamani S, Turner R, Mitchell C, Wade JB, Knepper MA. The thiazide-sensitive Na-Cl cotransporter is an aldosterone-induced protein. Proceedings of the National Academy of Sciences of the United States of America. 1998;**95**(24):14552-14557

[15] Young MJ, Moussa L, Dilley R, Funder JW. Early inflammatory responses in experimental cardiac hypertrophy and fibrosis: Effects of 11 beta-hydroxysteroid dehydrogenase inactivation. Endocrinology. 2003;**144**(3):1121-1125

[16] Sheppard KE, Autelitano DJ. 11Beta-hydroxysteroid dehydrogenase 1 transforms 11-dehydrocorticosterone into transcriptionally active glucocorticoid in neonatal rat heart. Endocrinology. 2002;**143**(1):198-204

[17] Tomaschitz A, Pilz S, Ritz E, Obermayer-Pietsch B, Pieber TR.

Aldosterone and arterial hypertension. Nature Reviews Endocrinology. 2010;**6**(2):83-93

[18] Young M, Funder JW. Aldosterone and the heart. Trends in Endocrinology and Metabolism. 2000;**11**(6):224-226

[19] Payne AH, Hales DB. Overview of steroidogenic enzymes in the pathway from cholesterol to active steroid hormones. Endocrine Reviews. 2004;**25**(6):947-970

[20] White PC, Curnow KM, Pascoe L. Disorders of steroid 11 beta-hydroxylase isozymes. Endocrine Reviews. 1994;**15**(4):421-438

[21] Gomez-Sanchez CE, Gomez-Sanchez EP. Immunohistochemistry of the adrenal in primary aldosteronism. Current Opinion in Endocrinology, Diabetes, and Obesity. 2016;**23**(3):242-248

[22] Miller WL, Bose HS. Early steps in steroidogenesis: Intracellular cholesterol trafficking. Journal of Lipid Research. 2011;**52**(12):2111-2135

[23] Dores RM, Londraville RL, Prokop J, Davis P, Dewey N, Lesinski N. Molecular evolution of GPCRs: Melanocortin/melanocortin receptors. Journal of Molecular Endocrinology. 2014;**52**(3):T29-T42

[24] El Ghorayeb N, Bourdeau I, Lacroix A. Role of ACTH and other hormones in the regulation of aldosterone production in primary aldosteronism. Frontiers in Endocrinology. 2016;**7**:72

[25] Evans JF, Fernando A, Ragolia L. Functional melanocortin-2 receptors are expressed by mouse aorta-derived mesenchymal progenitor cells. Molecular and Cellular Endocrinology. 2012;**355**(1):60-70

[26] Bassett MH, White PC, Rainey WE. The regulation of aldosterone synthase expression. Molecular and Cellular Endocrinology. 2004;**217**(1-2):67-74

[27] Shen Y, Xu L, Foster DA. Role for phospholipase D in receptor-mediated endocytosis. Molecular and Cellular Biology. 2001;**21**(2):595-602

[28] Condon JC, Pezzi V, Drummond BM, Yin S, Rainey WE. Calmodulin-dependent kinase I regulates adrenal cell expression of aldosterone synthase. Endocrinology. 2002;**143**(9):3651-3657

[29] Spat A, Hunyady L, Szanda G. Signaling interactions in the adrenal cortex. Frontiers in Endocrinology. 2016;**7**:17

[30] Spat A, Hunyady L. Control of aldosterone secretion: A model for convergence in cellular signaling pathways. Physiological Reviews. 2004;**84**(2):489-539

[31] Freel EM, Connell JM. Mechanisms of hypertension: The expanding role of aldosterone. Journal of the American Society of Nephrology. 2004;**15**(8):1993-2001

[32] Gomez-Sanchez CE, Oki K. Minireview: Potassium channels and aldosterone dysregulation: Is primary aldosteronism a potassium channelopathy? Endocrinology. 2014;**155**(1):47-55

[33] Bassett MH, Suzuki T, Sasano H, White PC, Rainey WE. The orphan nuclear receptors NURR1 and NGFIB regulate adrenal aldosterone production. Molecular Endocrinology. 2004;**18**(2):279-290

[34] Thiel G, Al Sarraj J, Vinson C, Stefano L, Bach K. Role of basic region leucine zipper transcription factors cyclic AMP response element binding protein (CREB), CREB2, activating transcription factor 2 and CAAT/enhancer binding protein alpha

in cyclic AMP response element-mediated transcription. Journal of Neurochemistry. 2005;**92**(2):321-336

[35] Naqvi S, Martin KJ, Arthur JS. CREB phosphorylation at Ser133 regulates transcription via distinct mechanisms downstream of cAMP and MAPK signalling. The Biochemical Journal. 2014;**458**(3):469-479

[36] Johannessen M, Delghandi MP, Seternes OM, Johansen B, Moens U. Synergistic activation of CREB-mediated transcription by forskolin and phorbol ester requires PKC and depends on the glutamine-rich Q2 transactivation domain. Cellular Signalling. 2004;**16**(10):1187-1199

[37] Cheng LC, Pai TW, Li LA. Regulation of human *CYP11B1* and *CYP11B2* promoters by transposable elements and conserved cis elements. Steroids. 2012;**77**(1-2):100-109

[38] Li W, Liu C. The −344C/T polymorphism in the *CYP11B2* gene is associated with essential hypertension in the Chinese. Journal of the Renin-Angiotensin-Aldosterone System. 2014;**15**(2):150-155

[39] Gardiner JR, Shima Y, Morohashi K, Swain A. SF-1 expression during adrenal development and tumourigenesis. Molecular and Cellular Endocrinology. 2012;**351**(1):12-18

[40] Suntharalingham JP, Buonocore F, Duncan AJ, Achermann JC. DAX-1 (NR0B1) and steroidogenic factor-1 (SF-1, NR5A1) in human disease. Best Practice & Research: Clinical Endocrinology & Metabolism. 2015;**29**(4):607-619

[41] Bassett MH, Zhang Y, Clyne C, White PC, Rainey WE. Differential regulation of aldosterone synthase and 11beta-hydroxylase transcription by steroidogenic factor-1. Journal of Molecular Endocrinology. 2002;**28**(2):125-135

[42] Shibata H, Ikeda Y, Mukai T, Morohashi K, Kurihara I, Ando T, et al. Expression profiles of COUP-TF, DAX-1, and SF-1 in the human adrenal gland and adrenocortical tumors: Possible implications in steroidogenesis. Molecular Genetics and Metabolism. 2001;**74**(1-2):206-216

[43] Vamsi UM, Swapna N, Padma G, Vishnupriya S, Padma T. Haplotype association and synergistic effect of human aldosterone synthase (*CYP11B2*) gene polymorphisms causing susceptibility to essential hypertension in Indian patients. Clinical and Experimental Hypertension. 2016;**38**(8):659-665

[44] White PC, Rainey WE. Editorial: Polymorphisms in *CYP11B* genes and 11-hydroxylase activity. The Journal of Clinical Endocrinology and Metabolism. 2005;**90**(2):1252-1255

[45] Nicod J, Bruhin D, Auer L, Vogt B, Frey FJ, Ferrari P. A biallelic gene polymorphism of *CYP11B2* predicts increased aldosterone to renin ratio in selected hypertensive patients. The Journal of Clinical Endocrinology and Metabolism. 2003;**88**(6):2495-2500

[46] Staessen JA, Wang JG, Brand E, Barlassina C, Birkenhager WH, Herrmann SM, et al. Effects of three candidate genes on prevalence and incidence of hypertension in a Caucasian population. Journal of Hypertension. 2001;**19**(8):1349-1358

[47] Lim PO, Macdonald TM, Holloway C, Friel E, Anderson NH, Dow E, et al. Variation at the aldosterone synthase (*CYP11B2*) locus contributes to hypertension in subjects with a raised aldosterone-to-renin ratio. The Journal of Clinical Endocrinology and Metabolism. 2002;**87**(9):4398-4402

[48] Sookoian S, Gianotti TF, Gonzalez CD, Pirola CJ. Association of

the C-344T aldosterone synthase gene variant with essential hypertension: A meta-analysis. Journal of Hypertension. 2007;**25**(1):5-13

[49] Ganapathipillai S, Laval G, Hoffmann IS, Castejon AM, Nicod J, Dick B, et al. *CYP11B2-CYP11B1* haplotypes associated with decreased 11 beta-hydroxylase activity. The Journal of Clinical Endocrinology and Metabolism. 2005;**90**(2):1220-1225

[50] Connell JM, Fraser R, MacKenzie S, Davies E. Is altered adrenal steroid biosynthesis a key intermediate phenotype in hypertension? Hypertension. 2003;**41**(5):993-999

[51] Keavney B, Mayosi B, Gaukrodger N, Imrie H, Baker M, Fraser R, et al. Genetic variation at the locus encompassing 11-beta hydroxylase and aldosterone synthase accounts for heritability in cortisol precursor (11-deoxycortisol) urinary metabolite excretion. The Journal of Clinical Endocrinology and Metabolism. 2005;**90**(2):1072-1077

[52] Tanahashi H, Mune T, Takahashi Y, Isaji M, Suwa T, Morita H, et al. Association of Lys173Arg polymorphism with *CYP11B2* expression in normal adrenal glands and aldosterone-producing adenomas. The Journal of Clinical Endocrinology and Metabolism. 2005;**90**(11):6226-6231

[53] Mayosi BM, Keavney B, Watkins H, Farrall M. Measured haplotype analysis of the aldosterone synthase gene and heart size. European Journal of Human Genetics. 2003;**11**(5):395-401

[54] Giles TD, Materson BJ, Cohn JN, Kostis JB. Definition and classification of hypertension: An update. Journal of Clinical Hypertension. 2009;**11**(11):611-614

[55] Sarkar T, Singh NP. Epidemiology and genetics of hypertension. The Journal of the Association of Physicians of India. 2015;**63**(9):61-98

[56] Padmanabhan S, Caulfield M, Dominiczak AF. Genetic and molecular aspects of hypertension. Circulation Research. 2015;**116**(6):937-959

[57] Rajput C, Arif E, Vibhuti A, Stobdan T, Khan AP, Norboo T, et al. Predominance of interaction among wild-type alleles of *CYP11B2* in Himalayan natives associates with high-altitude adaptation. Biochemical and Biophysical Research Communications. 2006;**348**(2):735-740

[58] Casiglia E, Tikhonoff V, Mazza A, Rynkiewicz A, Limon J, Caffi S, et al. C-344T polymorphism of the aldosterone synthase gene and blood pressure in the elderly: A population-based study. Journal of Hypertension. 2005;**23**(11):1991-1996

[59] Rajan S, Ramu P, Shewade DG, Adithan C. Promotor gene polymorphism of *CYP11B2* (344C>T) of healthy volunteer of south Indian tamilian population. Indian Journal of Biotechnology. 2009;**8**:358-362

[60] Sia SK, Chiou HL, Chen SC, Tsai CF, Yang SF, Ueng KC. Distribution and phenotypic expression of mineralocorticoid receptor and *CYP11B2* T-344C polymorphisms in a Taiwanese hypertensive population. Molecular Biology Reports. 2013;**40**(5):3705-3711

[61] Abdel Ghafar MT. Association of aldosterone synthase *CYP11B2* (−344C/T) gene polymorphism with essential hypertension and left ventricular hypertrophy in the Egyptian population. Clinical and Experimental Hypertension. 2019;**41**(8):779-786

[62] Tsukada K, Ishimitsu T, Teranishi M, Saitoh M, Yoshii M, Inada H, et al. Positive association of *CYP11B2* gene polymorphism with genetic

predisposition to essential hypertension. Journal of Human Hypertension. 2002;**16**(11):789-793

[63] Kumar NN, Benjafield AV, Lin RC, Wang WY, Stowasser M, Morris BJ. Haplotype analysis of aldosterone synthase gene (CYP11B2) polymorphisms shows association with essential hypertension. Journal of Hypertension. 2003;**21**(7):1331-1337

[64] Ji X, Qi H, Li DB, Liu RK, Zheng Y, Chen HL, et al. Associations between human aldosterone synthase *CYP11B2* (−344T/C) gene polymorphism and antihypertensive response to valsartan in Chinese patients with essential hypertension. International Journal of Clinical and Experimental Medicine. 2015;**8**(1):1173-1177

[65] Li X, Xie P, He J, Cai H, Yang R, Zhang Q, et al. *CYP11B2* gene polymorphism and essential hypertension among Tibetan, Dongxiang and Han populations from northwest of China. Clinical and Experimental Hypertension. 2016;**38**(4):375-380

[66] Cheng X, Xu G. Association between aldosterone synthase *CYP11B2* polymorphism and essential hypertension in Chinese: A meta-analysis. Kidney & Blood Pressure Research. 2009;**32**(2):128-140

[67] Tsujita Y, Iwai N, Katsuya T, Higaki J, Ogihara T, Tamaki S, et al. Lack of association between genetic polymorphism of *CYP11B2* and hypertension in Japanese: The Suita study. Hypertension Research. 2001;**24**(2):105-109

[68] Chen JF, Jing J, Tan H, Song MB, Yu SY, Huang L. Lack of association of *CYP11B2*-344C/T polymorphism with essential hypertension: A meta-analysis. International Journal of Clinical and Experimental Medicine. 2015;8(6):9162-9167

[69] Zhu H, Sagnella GA, Dong Y, Miller MA, Onipinla A, Markandu ND, et al. Contrasting associations between aldosterone synthase gene polymorphisms and essential hypertension in blacks and in whites. Journal of Hypertension. 2003;**21**(1):87-95

[70] Yu H, Lin S, Zhang Y, Liu G. Intron-2 conversion polymorphism of the aldosterone synthase gene and the antihypertensive response to angiotensin-converting enzyme inhibitors. Journal of Hypertension. 2008;**26**(2):251-256

[71] Fox CS, Parise H, D'Agostino RB Sr, Lloyd-Jones DM, Vasan RS, Wang TJ, et al. Parental atrial fibrillation as a risk factor for atrial fibrillation in offspring. JAMA. 2004;**291**(23):2851-2855

[72] Tsai CT, Lai LP, Hwang JJ, Lin JL, Chiang FT. Molecular genetics of atrial fibrillation. Journal of the American College of Cardiology. 2008;**52**(4):241-250

[73] Tsai CT, Lai LP, Lin JL, Chiang FT, Hwang JJ, Ritchie MD, et al. Renin-angiotensin system gene polymorphisms and atrial fibrillation. Circulation. 2004;**109**(13):1640-1646

[74] Amir O, Amir RE, Paz H, Mor R, Sagiv M, Lewis BS. Aldosterone synthase gene polymorphism as a determinant of atrial fibrillation in patients with heart failure. The American Journal of Cardiology. 2008;**102**(3):326-329

[75] Lu WH, Bayike M, Liu JW, Wang S, Xie X, Yang YC, et al. Association between aldosterone synthase (*CYP11B2*) −344C/T polymorphism and atrial fibrillation among Han and Kazak residents of the Xinjiang region. International Journal of Clinical and Experimental Medicine. 2015;**8**(4):5513-5519

[76] Li YY, Zhou CW, Xu J, Qian Y, Wang B. *CYP11B2* T-344C gene

polymorphism and atrial fibrillation: A meta-analysis of 2,758 subjects. PLoS One. 2012;**7**(11):e50910

[77] Zhang XL, Wu LQ, Liu X, Yang YQ, Tan HW, Wang XH, et al. Association of angiotensin-converting enzyme gene I/D and *CYP11B2* gene −344T/C polymorphisms with lone atrial fibrillation and its recurrence after catheter ablation. Experimental and Therapeutic Medicine. 2012;**4**(4):741-747

[78] Niu W, Qi Y, Hou S, Zhai X, Zhou W, Qiu C. Haplotype-based association of the renin-angiotensin-aldosterone system genes polymorphisms with essential hypertension among Han Chinese: The Fangshan study. Journal of Hypertension. 2009;**27**(7):1384-1391

[79] Boos CJ, Anderson RA, Lip GY. Is atrial fibrillation an inflammatory disorder? European Heart Journal. 2006;**27**(2):136-149

[80] Dixen U, Ravn L, Soeby-Rasmussen C, Paulsen AW, Parner J, Frandsen E, et al. Raised plasma aldosterone and natriuretic peptides in atrial fibrillation. Cardiology. 2007;**108**(1):35-39

[81] Sekuri C, Cam FS, Ercan E, Tengiz I, Sagcan A, Eser E, et al. Renin-angiotensin system gene polymorphisms and premature coronary heart disease. Journal of the Renin-Angiotensin-Aldosterone System. 2005;**6**(1):38-42

[82] Franco E, Palumbo L, Crobu F, Anselmino M, Frea S, Matullo G, et al. Renin-angiotensin-aldosterone system polymorphisms: A role or a hole in occurrence and long-term prognosis of acute myocardial infarction at young age. BMC Medical Genetics. 2007;**8**:27

[83] Liu Y, Liu HL, Han W, Yu SJ, Zhang J. Association between the *CYP11B2* gene −344T>C polymorphism and coronary artery disease: A meta-analysis. Genetics and Molecular Research. 2015;**14**(2):3121-3128

[84] Chou CH, Ueng KC, Yang SF, Wu CH, Wang PH. Relationship of genetic polymorphisms of aldosterone synthase gene cytochrome P450 11B2 and mineralocorticoid receptors with coronary artery disease in Taiwan. International Journal of Medical Sciences. 2016;**13**(2):117-123

[85] Sharma R, Katz J. Preliminary studies on human aldosterone synthase (*CYP11B2*) gene polymorphism, matrix metalloprotease-9, apoptosis, and carotid atherosclerosis plaque size by proton magnetic resonance imaging. Journal of the Renin-Angiotensin-Aldosterone System. 2010;**11**(3):198-204

[86] Padmanabhan N, Padmanabhan S, Connell JM. Genetic basis of cardiovascular disease--the renin-angiotensin-aldosterone system as a paradigm. Journal of the Renin-Angiotensin-Aldosterone System. 2000;**1**(4):316-324

[87] Borzyszkowska J, Stanislawska-Sachadyn A, Wirtwein M, Sobiczewski W, Ciecwierz D, Targonski R, et al. Angiotensin converting enzyme gene polymorphism is associated with severity of coronary artery disease in men with high total cholesterol levels. Journal of Applied Genetics. 2012;**53**(2):175-182

[88] Mishra A, Srivastava A, Mittal T, Garg N, Mittal B. Impact of renin-angiotensin-aldosterone system gene polymorphisms on left ventricular dysfunction in coronary artery disease patients. Disease Markers. 2012;**32**(1):33-41

[89] Sarzani R, Salvi F, Dessi-Fulgheri P, Catalini R, Mazzara D, Cola G, et al. Aldosterone synthase alleles and cardiovascular phenotype in young

adults. Journal of Human Hypertension. 2003;**17**(12):859-864

[90] Jia EZ, Xu ZX, Guo CY, Li L, Gu Y, Zhu TB, et al. Renin-angiotensin-aldosterone system gene polymorphisms and coronary artery disease: Detection of gene-gene and gene-environment interactions. Cellular Physiology and Biochemistry. 2012;**29**(3-4):443-452

[91] Hautanen A, Toivanen P, Manttari M, Tenkanen L, Kupari M, Manninen V, et al. Joint effects of an aldosterone synthase (*CYP11B2*) gene polymorphism and classic risk factors on risk of myocardial infarction. Circulation. 1999;**100**(22):2213-2218

[92] Ommen SR, Nishimura RA. Hypertrophic cardiomyopathy. Current Problems in Cardiology. 2004;**29**(5):239-291

[93] Tsybouleva N, Zhang L, Chen S, Patel R, Lutucuta S, Nemoto S, et al. Aldosterone, through novel signaling proteins, is a fundamental molecular bridge between the genetic defect and the cardiac phenotype of hypertrophic cardiomyopathy. Circulation. 2004;**109**(10):1284-1291

[94] Bureik M, Hubel K, Dragan CA, Scher J, Becker H, Lenz N, et al. Development of test systems for the discovery of selective human aldosterone synthase (*CYP11B2*) and 11beta-hydroxylase (*CYP11B1*) inhibitors. Discovery of a new lead compound for the therapy of congestive heart failure, myocardial fibrosis and hypertension. Molecular and Cellular Endocrinology. 2004;**217**(1-2):249-254

[95] Yoshida Y, Morimoto T, Takaya T, Kawamura T, Sunagawa Y, Wada H, et al. Aldosterone signaling associates with p300/GATA4 transcriptional pathway during the hypertrophic response of cardiomyocytes. Circulation Journal. 2010;**74**(1):156-162

[96] Kupari M, Hautanen A, Lankinen L, Koskinen P, Virolainen J, Nikkila H, et al. Associations between human aldosterone synthase (*CYP11B2*) gene polymorphisms and left ventricular size, mass, and function. Circulation. 1998;**97**(6):569-575

[97] Chai W, Hoedemaekers Y, van Schaik RH, van Fessem M, Garrelds IM, Saris JJ, et al. Cardiac aldosterone in subjects with hypertrophic cardiomyopathy. Journal of the Renin-Angiotensin-Aldosterone System. 2006;**7**(4):225-230

[98] Ortlepp JR, Vosberg HP, Reith S, Ohme F, Mahon NG, Schroder D, et al. Genetic polymorphisms in the renin-angiotensin-aldosterone system associated with expression of left ventricular hypertrophy in hypertrophic cardiomyopathy: A study of five polymorphic genes in a family with a disease causing mutation in the myosin binding protein C gene. Heart. 2002;**87**(3):270-275

[99] Perkins MJ, Van Driest SL, Ellsworth EG, Will ML, Gersh BJ, Ommen SR, et al. Gene-specific modifying effects of pro-LVH polymorphisms involving the renin-angiotensin-aldosterone system among 389 unrelated patients with hypertrophic cardiomyopathy. European Heart Journal. 2005;**26**(22):2457-2462

[100] Ortlepp JR, Breithardt O, Ohme F, Hanrath P, Hoffmann R. Lack of association among five genetic polymorphisms of the renin-angiotensin system and cardiac hypertrophy in patients with aortic stenosis. American Heart Journal. 2001;**141**(4):671-676

[101] Schunkert H, Hengstenberg C, Holmer SR, Broeckel U, Luchner A, Muscholl MW, et al. Lack of association between a polymorphism of the aldosterone synthase gene and left ventricular structure. Circulation. 1999;**99**(17):2255-2260

[102] Bleumink GS, Schut AF, Sturkenboom MC, Deckers JW, van Duijn CM, Stricker BH. Genetic polymorphisms and heart failure. Genetics in Medicine. 2004;**6**(6):465-474

[103] Kaufman BD, Auerbach S, Reddy S, Manlhiot C, Deng L, Prakash A, et al. RAAS gene polymorphisms influence progression of pediatric hypertrophic cardiomyopathy. Human Genetics. 2007;**122**(5):515-523

[104] Kitzman DW, Little WC, Brubaker PH, Anderson RT, Hundley WG, Marburger CT, et al. Pathophysiological characterization of isolated diastolic heart failure in comparison to systolic heart failure. JAMA. 2002;**288**(17):2144-2150

[105] McMurray JJ, Pfeffer MA. Heart failure. Lancet. 2005;**365**(9474):1877-1889

[106] Swedberg K, Cleland J, Dargie H, Drexler H, Follath F, Komajda M, et al. Guidelines for the diagnosis and treatment of chronic heart failure: Executive summary (update 2005). The Task Force for the Diagnosis and Treatment of Chronic Heart Failure of the European Society of Cardiology. European Heart Journal. 2005;**26**(11):1115-1140

[107] Muthumala A, Drenos F, Elliott PM, Humphries SE. Role of beta adrenergic receptor polymorphisms in heart failure: Systematic review and meta-analysis. European Journal of Heart Failure. 2008;**10**(1):3-13

[108] McNamara DM, Tam SW, Sabolinski ML, Tobelmann P, Janosko K, Taylor AL, et al. Aldosterone synthase promoter polymorphism predicts outcome in African Americans with heart failure: Results from the A-HeFT Trial. Journal of the American College of Cardiology. 2006;**48**(6):1277-1282

[109] Feola M, Monteverde M, Vivenza D, Testa M, Leto L, Astesana V, et al. Prognostic value of different allelic polymorphism of aldosterone synthase receptor in a congestive heart failure European continental ancestry population. Archives of Medical Research. 2017;**48**(2):156-161

[110] Tiago AD, Badenhorst D, Skudicky D, Woodiwiss AJ, Candy GP, Brooksbank R, et al. An aldosterone synthase gene variant is associated with improvement in left ventricular ejection fraction in dilated cardiomyopathy. Cardiovascular Research. 2002;**54**(3):584-589

[111] Biolo A, Chao T, Duhaney TA, Kotlyar E, Allensworth-Davies D, Loscalzo J, et al. Usefulness of the aldosterone synthase gene polymorphism C−344-T to predict cardiac remodeling in African-Americans versus non-African-Americans with chronic systolic heart failure. The American Journal of Cardiology. 2007;**100**(2):285-290

[112] Bress A, Han J, Patel SR, Desai AA, Mansour I, Groo V, et al. Association of aldosterone synthase polymorphism (*CYP11B2* −344T>C) and genetic ancestry with atrial fibrillation and serum aldosterone in African Americans with heart failure. PLoS One. 2013;**8**(7):e71268

Chapter 3

Single-Nucleotide Polymorphisms in Inflammatory Bowel Disease

Ewa Dudzińska

Abstract

Inflammatory bowel disease (IBD) mainly includes ulcerative colitis (UC) and Crohn's disease (CD). Both conditions are characterized by chronic inflammation of the gastrointestinal tract, with alternating periods of relapse and remission. Both forms of IBD involve an uncontrolled inflammatory process in the intestines, leading to worsening quality of life and requiring long-term medical and/or surgical intervention. Epidemiological and clinical studies suggest that the pathogenesis of inflammatory bowel disease is strongly linked to genetic predisposition. CD and UC are considered polygenic diseases in which familial clustering is observed in 5–10% of patients. Among genetic factors associated with IBD development, it has been found that many single nucleotide polymorphisms are associated with susceptibility to IBD progression. SNP can affect the production or function of a protein and thus affect the development of the disease. However, although the overall role of genes involved in the development of IBD is already in most cases known, as of today it is unclear how the SNPs in these genes affect cellular function, or how such changed cellular functions would contribute to the development of IBD. In the present work several selected polymorphisms in genes involved in IBD development are discussed.

Keywords: ulcerative colitis, Crohn's disease, single-nucleotide polymorphisms

1. Introduction

Inflammatory bowel disease (IBD) mainly includes ulcerative colitis (UC) and Crohn's disease (CD). Both conditions are characterized by chronic inflammation of the gastrointestinal tract, with alternating periods of relapse and remission. Both forms of IBD involve an uncontrolled inflammatory process in the intestines, leading to worsening quality of life and requiring long-term medical and/or surgical intervention [1].

The pathomechanism of IBD is still not well explain, but evidence suggests that it results from perturbation of the homeostasis between the intestinal microbiota and the mucosal immune system, with the involvement of both genetic and environmental factors [2].

Ulcerative colitis is a chronic inflammatory disease, which mainly affects the large intestine. Typical clinical symptoms of UC are diarrhea, rectal bleeding, and abdominal pain. Nonspecific symptoms include fever, appetite loss, and weight loss. The disease significantly affects the patient's quality of life due to its repeated remissions and relapses [3].

UC is characterized by recurring episodes of inflammation limited to the mucosal layer of the colon and practically invariably involves the rectum and may extend in a proximal and continuous fashion to involve other portions of the colon. Endoscopic features of inflammation include loss of vascular markings, granularity and friability of the mucosa, and erosions. In the setting of severe inflammation is observed deep ulcerations and spontaneous bleeding [4] (**Figure 1**). CD is described by transmural rather than superficial mucosal inflammation and by skip lesions rather than continuous disease [5].

In Crohn's disease, inflammatory changes may occur in all parts of the gastrointestinal tract, from the oral cavity to the rectum, but are usually localized in the terminal segment of the small intestine, that is, the ileum. Inflammatory changes are discontinuous and affect the entire thickness of the intestinal wall. The most common symptoms of CD are abdominal pain, fever, weight loss, and diarrhea [6].

The commonly used instrument for evaluating the disease severity of CD is Crohn's Disease Activity Indicator (CDAI; remission <150 score, severe disease >450 score). Whereas the Mayo score (0—normal, 3—severe disease) is used to assess the severity of ulcerative colitis [7].

The optimal goal of management in IBD is a durable period of steroid-free remission and the induction and subsequent maintenance of mucosal healing [4]. Mucosal healing is predominantly defined by endoscopic assessment of intestinal inflammation and is referred to as the absence of mucosal ulcerations in CD, while in UC, an international consensus defined it as the absence of friability, blood, erosions, and ulcers of the gut mucosa. However, these indices allow to determine improvements of endoscopic lesions, even when the rather rigid endpoint of mucosal healing, and thereby the total disappearance of all mucosal ulcerations is not met [8] (**Figure 2**).

Many genes, which may be linked to IBD, are believed to be associated with microbiological defense mechanisms involving the epithelial barrier and innate, adaptive immune systems [9].

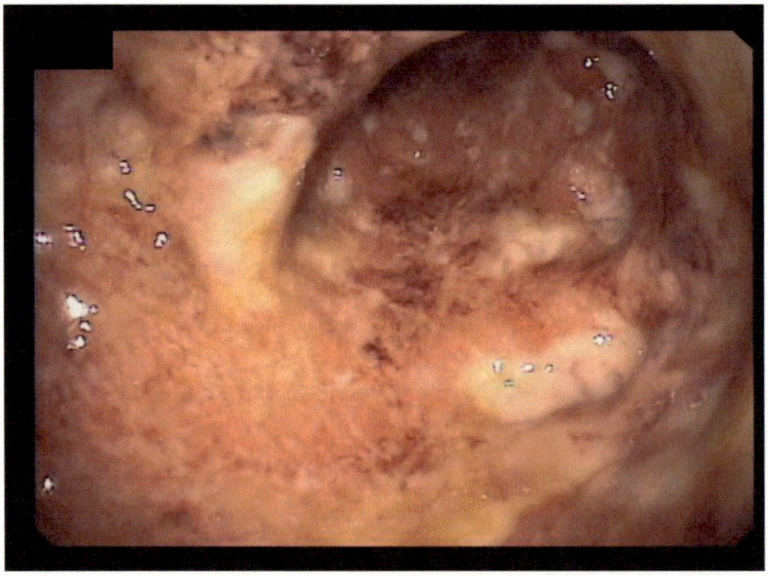

Figure 1.
Endoscopic images of ulcerative colitis according to the Mayo score (Grade 3—severe disease). (Source: Own study.)

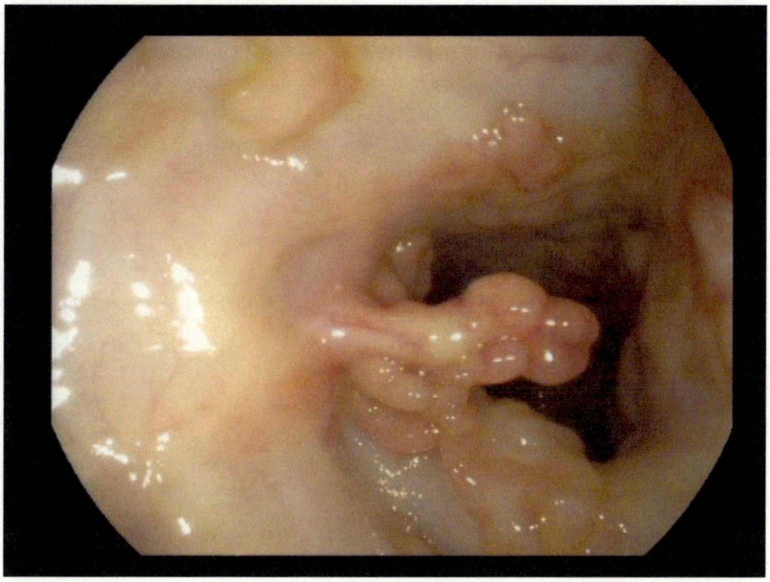

Figure 2.
Endoscopic assessment of the large intestine was observed by mucosal bridging and pseudopolyps, which confirms regeneration of the mucosa in the course of remission of ulcerative colitis. (Source: Own study.)

In the result of large cohort genome-wide association studies (GWAS) of cases and controls, over 200 IBD susceptibility loci have now been reported [10].

GWAS research was aimed at searching the SNPs that are over-represented in IBD patients when compared with healthy controls. SNPs that occurred more frequently in IBD patients are thus called disease-associated variants [11].

Among the genetic factors involved, there are several single-nucleotide polymorphisms (SNP) associated with the susceptibility to IBD progression. Many of these mutations regulate immune responses with several being enriched in immune cells, in particular CD4+ T cells and dendritic cells [12].

2. Single-nucleotide polymorphisms in innate and adaptive immunity genes in IBD

The latest research on genetics and immunology has confirmed that the innate immune system is of great importance in inducing intestinal inflammation [13], and the publication of Dudzińska et al. [14], "Single nucleotide polymorphisms in selected genes in inflammatory bowel disease," is dedicated to this issue. This paper attempts to demonstrate polymorphisms *NOD2/CARD15* (*nucleotide-binding oligomerization domain containing 2/caspase recruitment domain family number 15*) and the *DLG5* gene (*discs large homolog 5*) in patients with IBD hospitalized at the Department of Gastroenterology, Regional Specialist Hospital, SPZOZ im. Stefan Cardinal Wyszynski in Lublin.

NOD2/CARD15 is located on chromosome 16q12.1 and was the first disease-susceptibility gene discovered for CD. *NOD2/CARD15* is a pattern-recognition receptor that is involved in the homeostasis of intestinal immunity [15].

CARD15/NOD2 plays an important role in immune function. In response to bacterial infection, *CARD15/NOD2* acts as an intracellular bacterial receptor and activates the kappa B nuclear factor (NF-κB), particularly after recognizing the bacterial wall component muramyl dipeptide (MDP) [16].

NOD2/CARD15 mutations lead to dysregulation of host-microbe interactions, contributing to the development of inflammation in the ileum, which is characteristic of CD [17].

Today more than 60 polymorphisms of this gene have been identified; however, three common mutations Leu1007fsinsC, Arg702Trp, and Gly908Arg have been specifically associated with ileal involvement, stricturing complications, and earlier age of onset [18].

While the gene *DLG5* encodes scaffold proteins belonging to the MAGUK family, which participate in the formation of cellular connections, maintenance of cell shape, and intracellular signal transduction [19]. Expression of this gene is widely expressed in the tissues of the small and large intestines. *DLG5* gene polymorphisms have been shown to increase susceptibility to IBD, including both CD and UC [20]. *DLG5* has been shown to be localized at cell-cell contact sites and is involved in maintaining epithelial integrity. Different variants of *DLG5* may contribute to the loss of cell polarization complexes and adhesion complexes, so that epithelial cell polarity is not maintained, and epithelial-mesenchymal transition (EMT) is induced [20]. EMT is a process involving the transformation of immobile, polarized cells with an epithelial phenotype into cells with a mesenchymal phenotype. The characteristic features of EMT include lack of polarity and cell adhesion, reduced expression of E-cadherin, and increased mobility and invasion capacity [21].

Thus, it can be assumed that *DLG5* polymorphisms may impair the epithelial barrier in the gastrointestinal tract and lead to abnormal epithelial structure, making it more susceptible to IBD (CD and UC). Furthermore, the *DLG5* scaffold protein also belongs to the CARD family of proteins (like *CARD15/NOD2*). Thus, *DLG5* is probably involved in the regulation of NF-κB activation or caspase activation within the host defense mechanisms [22]. Therefore, both the *NOD2* and *DLG5* genes may interact functionally to contribute to the risk of developing CD.

Our research in the group of patients diagnosed with CD and UC is related to the occurrence of polymorphisms in the *NOD2* and *DLG5* genes.

The test material was blood collected from patients on an empty stomach after 12 hours of rest. In addition, medical history was taken with regard to the occurrence of extraintestinal symptoms and autoimmune diseases in the family. The family history of all subjects was negative. DNA was isolated using a QIAamp DNA Blood Mini Kit (QIAgen), followed by quantitative and qualitative evaluation of the isolated DNA samples.

The following primers were used for PCR: (F) GACTCTTTTGGCCTTTTCAGATT and (R) CCAATGGTCTTTTTTCCTTACTCC for *CARD15/NOD2* and (F) TTATTCCCCTTCCACAGGCACTAC and (R) GCCGCAGCTGAATGGAGA for *DLG5*.

The PCR product was sequenced, and the sequences obtained were recorded in FASTA format. The nucleotide sequences of the *CARD15/NOD2* and *DLG5* gene fragments were compared using DNA Baser software.

The size of the analyzed *CARD15/NOD2* gene fragment was 243 bp. No SNPs were observed in this fragment in patients with CD or UC.

Although numerous reports confirm that *CARD15/NOD2* gene polymorphisms are associated with a predisposition to IBD [23], our research did not show this relationship. This may be linked to the absence of parenteral symptoms in the subjects.

One of the most common single-nucleotide polymorphisms of the *CARD15/NOD2* gene is P268S (SNP5), where the cytosine residue at position 802 is replaced by thymine. In the Polish population, P268S polymorphism has been found in 49.5% of patients with CD, and its presence in both alleles is associated with earlier

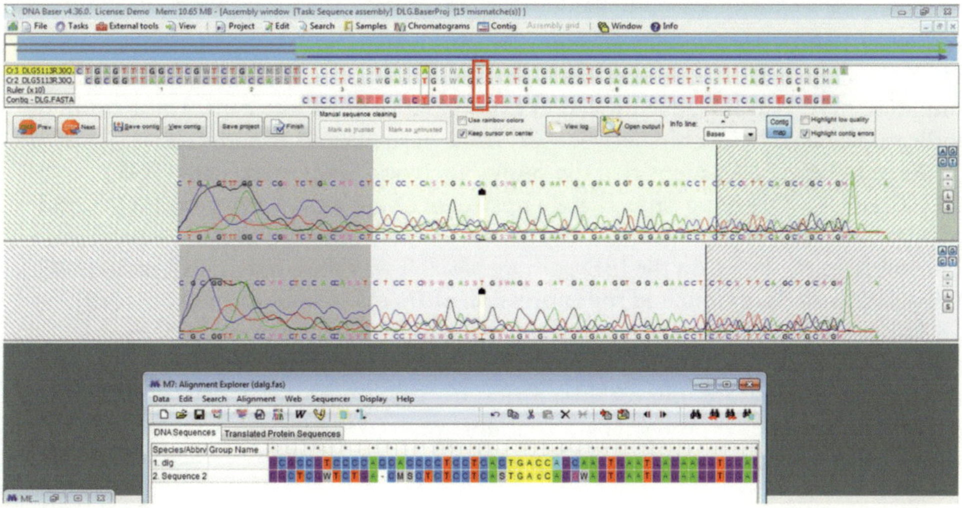

Figure 3.
SNP at position rs1248696, T > C substitution in a patient with Crohn's disease (source: Dudzińska et al. 2018).

onset of disease symptoms and increased risk of parenteral symptoms such as joint abnormalities, iritis, and erythema nodosum [24].

The size of the *DLG5* gene fragment was 107 bp. One SNP at position 1,248,696 was found in the gene fragment. A T > C substitution occurred in one sample (Patient 3) from the group of patients with Crohn's disease (**Figure 3**). Other authors note that the R30Q (Rs1248696) variant of *DLG5*, where amino acid 30 in exon 3 changes from arginine to glutamine, is associated with the development of IBD [25].

Despite numerous reports indicating the presence of polymorphisms of the *NOD2/CARD15* gene, our studies did not show the position of SNP in patients with IBD from the Lublin region. The study suggests that SNPs (T > C substitution) affect the function of the *DLG5* protein and thus play a role in the development of IBD, in particular Crohn's disease.

3. The role of autophagy genes in the pathogenesis of IBD

Autophagy is a conserved lysosome-dependent catabolic process, degrading and recycling protein aggregates or damaged organelle. Autophagy affects the pathogenesis of IBD in multiple ways, including secretion of antimicrobial materials from Paneth cells, clearance of invading pathogens, presentation of antigen, or proinflammatory cytokine production by macrophages [26].

SNPs of autophagy genes such as autophagy-related gene 16 like 1 (*ATG16L1*) and immunity-related GTPase family M (*IRGM*) have been identified to be associated with CD. *ATG16L1* and *IRGM* genes affect cellular autophagy processes and bacterial clearance in immune cells and may affect bacterial composition of the gut in patients with IBD [27].

There is some overlap in these autophagy-related genetic variants in both CD and UC, but majority of the identified variants are more associated with ileal CD. Despite this association, the positive predictive value for disease development in individuals carrying autophagy variants is low because the *ATG16L1* T300A polymorphism is linked with CD susceptibility, which is also present in a large proportion of healthy individuals who do not develop IBD [28].

However, some of the studies show that a knock-in mouse model expressing *ATG16L1* T300A does not develop spontaneous inflammation, but it exhibits morphological defects in both Paneth cells and goblet cells, and the presence of the T300A mutation in *ATG16L1* leads to aberrant functionality of Paneth cells. These findings indicate a close relationship between *ATG16L1* variants and Paneth cells [15].

Recent data GWAS identified the single-nucleotide polymorphism (SNP) rs13361189—a SNP lying immediately upstream of the autophagy gene *IRGM*, and many studies have investigated *IRGM* gene variants both in adult and pediatric and in UC, confirming its role in the IBD pathogenesis. It was shown that SNP rs13361189, the deletion allele, modulated the expression of *IRGM* in transformed cells [29].

Other study demonstrated functional effects of the synonymous SNP rs10065172 (c.313C > T). This synonymous variant rs10065172 in *IRGM* alters a binding site for certain microRNAs, miR-196, and causes deregulation of *IRGM*-dependent xenophagy of bacteria in patients with CD [29].

4. AHR and its role in regulating intestinal inflammation

Tryptophan metabolism plays important roles in the pathogenesis and therapeutics of IBD [30]. Recent study investigates the interaction between Card9 and the gut microbiota in the generation of the microbiota-derived tryptophan metabolite [2].

Tryptophan can be metabolized either by the gut bacteria into indole derivatives, such as indole-3-acetic acid (IAA), or by host cells into kynurenine (Kyn) via indoleamine 2,3-dioxygenase 1 (IDO1) [31].

Kyn derived from host metabolism, and indole-derived tryptophan metabolites produced by gut microbiota are endogenous ligands of aryl hydrocarbon receptor (AHR), an important regulator of immune response. AHR disturbance results in disordered immune responses, including decreased Treg cell levels and increased TNF-α levels, and a modified timeframe of IL-10 and IL-12 secretion. Elevated the serum levels of tryptophan metabolites including kynurenic acid (KA) is potential aryl hydrocarbon receptor (AHR) ligands to impact colitis. Several findings suggest that KA and other tryptophan metabolites inhibit the colonic inflammation [30].

Although polymorphisms in AHR have not yet been associated with IBD, AHR is known to play a central role in the regulation of intestinal inflammation and is upregulated in the inflamed gut [12].

SNPs are common, single-nucleotide genetic variants that can influence protein function, protein stability, or gene expression. Genome-wide association studies and candidate gene studies have identified SNPs near AHR target genes that are significantly associated with AHR-regulated phenotypes, such as psoriasis (CYP1A1) and systemic lupus erythematous (CYP1A1). These findings suggest that SNPs near AHR-binding sites might impact AHR target gene expression and contribute to individual variation in disease risk and pharmacotherapy phenotypes. Of interest, that SNP is distant from an AHR response element (AHRE) but still influences AHR binding and CYP1A1 expression after AHR agonist treatment, which suggests that it may influence the stability of the AHR complex and its ability to regulate CYP1A1 gene expression [32].

It is also important that over the last years, some functions of noncoding DNA have been discovered, and the role of regulatory sequences in transcriptional regulation, development of the disease process, and determination of cell type specificity is nowadays widely appreciated [11].

In the latest research, Boyd et al. [33] presented Cap Analysis of Gene Expression (CAGE) analysis on biopsies from the descending colon from 94 IBD patients and controls. These data enabled annotation of IBD-regulated enhancers and transcription start sites (TSSs) and characterization of IBD-associated

SNPs in such regions. Researchers have shown that clear overrepresentation of IBD-associated SNPs in both IBD upregulated enhancer and promoter regions also presented regions that had the largest IBD heritability enrichment compared to other genomic regions. The results of these studies carried out many resources for interpretation of the functional impact of noncoding genetic variants [33].

5. SNPs in the multi-drug resistance 1 gene

Another of the genes whose mutations may play a role in the pathogenesis of IBD is multi-drug resistance 1 (*MDR1*) gene. *MDR1* encodes P-glycoprotein 170 (P-gp), an ATP-dependent drug transport efflux pump, which highly expressed in many cells and epithelial surfaces, including the epithelium of GI tract [34].

In the gut, P-gp is expressed on the apical surfaces of the superficial columnar epithelial cells in the intestine with the levels of expression gradually rising from the duodenum to the distal parts of the intestine with the highest levels of expression in the distal small bowel and colon [35].

It is now known that substrates for the P-gp pump include a variety of structurally and pharmacologically distinct hydrophobic compounds, such as drugs and toxins, and P-gp might also play a critical role in host bacterial interactions in the gastrointestinal tract and maintenance of intestinal homeostasis [34].

SNPs of *MDR1* can occur naturally in humans, but some of them were related to altered P-gp expression and function. Three most common SNPs that have been repeatedly shown to predict changes in the function of P-gp are synonymous SNPs C1236T (rs1128503) in exon 12 and C3435T (rs1045642) in exon 26 and nonsynonymous, triallelic SNP G2677T/A (Ala893Ser/Thr or rs2032582) located in exon 21. In German, studies have been shown that both T allele and TT genotype of C3435T polymorphism were more frequently present among UC subjects, and the association of G allele of 2677 and IBD was also shown in North American study. However, further research that analyzed different allele combinations of those SNPs in IBD patients gave conflicting results [34].

6. SNPs in the neutrophil cytosolic factor 4 gene

More recently, GWAS has identified a number of new genetic susceptibility factors for IBD. Of these, new candidates have confirmed the association of the proinflammatory cytokine interleukin-23 receptor subunit (IL-23R) with CD and UC and a second gene, neutrophil cytosolic factor 4 (*NCF4*) with CD [36].

Researchers, Nuij et al. [27], have demonstrated that an IBD-associated SNP in the neutrophil cytosolic factor 4 (*NCF4*) gene results in a decreased antimicrobial function of granulocytes, as demonstrated by a reduced production of reactive oxygen species by these cells [27]. Moreover, as recently shown, SNPs in the interleukin 23 receptor gene (IL23R) have affected to express the anti-microbial peptide DMBT1 in intestinal epithelial cells in IBD [27].

7. Conclusion

Chronic inflammatory bowel disease is a subject of great interest among researchers because the pathomechanism of these conditions is difficult to explain, and thus far there is no optimal therapeutic process completely eliminating the symptoms and effects of the disease [37, 38].

Epidemiological and clinical studies suggest that the pathogenesis of inflammatory bowel disease is strongly linked to genetic predisposition [39, 40].

CD and UC are considered polygenic diseases in which familial clustering is observed in 5–10% of patients [41].

Among genetic factors associated with IBD development, it has been found that many single-nucleotide polymorphisms are associated with susceptibility to IBD progression. SNP can affect the production or function of a protein and thus affect the development of the disease [14].

However, although the overall role of genes involved in the development of IBD is already in most cases known, as of today it is unclear how the SNPs in these genes affect cellular function, or how such changed cellular functions would contribute to the development of IBD [27]. Therefore, further research is needed to demonstrate how gene polymorphism leads to the development of IBD.

Author details

Ewa Dudzińska
Medical University of Lublin, Poland

*Address all correspondence to: ewadudzinska@umlub.pl

References

[1] Vezza T, Rodríguez-Nogales A, Algieri F, et al. Flavonoids in inflammatory bowel disease: A review. Nutrients. 2016;**8**:211

[2] Etienne-Mesmin L, Chassaing B, Gewirtz AT. Tryptophan: A gut microbiota-derived metabolites regulating inflammation. World Journal of Gastrointestinal Pharmacology and Therapeutics. 2017;**8**(1):7-9. DOI: 10.4292/wjgpt.v8.i1.7

[3] Lan D, Niu J, Miao J, Dong X, Wang H, Yang G, et al. Expression of guanylate cyclase-C, guanylin, and uroguanylin is downregulated proportionally to the ulcerative colitis disease activity index. Scientific Reports. 2016;**6**:25034. DOI: 10.1038/srep25034

[4] Rubin DT, Ananthakrishnan AN, Siegel CA, Sauer BG, Long MD. ACG Clinical Guideline: Ulcerative colitis in adults. The American Journal of Gastroenterology. 2019;**114**(3):384-413. DOI: 10.14309/ajg.0000000000000152

[5] Agouridis AP, Elisaf M, Milionis HJ. An overview of lipid abnormalities in patients with inflammatory bowel disease. Annals of Gastroenterology. 2011;**24**(3):181-187

[6] Mahdi BM. Role of HLA typing on Crohn's disease pathogenesis. Annals of Medicine and Surgery. 2015;**4**:248-253

[7] Dudzińska E, Szymona K, Gil-Kulik P, Chomik P, Świstowska M, Gryzińska M, et al. Imbalance of controlled death in peripheral blood lymphocytes in Crohn's disease and ulcerative colitis. Medicina (Kaunas, Lithuania). 2019;**55**(6):231. DOI: 10.3390/medicina55060231

[8] Atreya R, Neurath MF. Current and future targets for mucosal healing in inflammatory bowel disease. Visceral Medicine. 2017;**33**(1):82-88. DOI: 10.1159/000458006

[9] Lee A, Kanuri N, Zhang Y, et al. IDO1 and IDO2 non-synonymous gene variants: Correlation with crohn's disease risk and clinical phenotype. PLoS One. 2014;**9**:115848

[10] Kennedy NA, Lamb CA, Berry SH, Walker AW, Mansfield J, Parkes M, et al. The impact of NOD2 variants on fecal microbiota in Crohn's disease and controls without gastrointestinal disease. Inflammatory Bowel Diseases. 2018;**24**(3):583-592. DOI: 10.1093/ibd/izx061

[11] Meddens CA, van der List ACJ, Nieuwenhuis EES, Mokry M. Non-coding DNA in IBD: From sequence variation in DNA regulatory elements to novel therapeutic potential. Gut. 2019;**68**:928-941

[12] Goettel JA, Gandhi R, Kenison JE, Yeste A, Murugaiyan G, Sambanthamoorthy S, et al. AHR activation is protective against colitis driven by T cells in humanized mice. Cell Reports. 2016;**17**(5):1318-1329. DOI: 10.1016/j.celrep.2016.09.082

[13] Bosca-Watts MM, Tosca J, Anton R, Mora M, Minguez M, Mora F. Pathogenesis of Crohn's disease: Bug or no bug. World Journal of Gastrointestinal Pathophysiology. 2015;**6**(1):1-12

[14] Dudzińska E, Gryzinska M, Kocki J. Single nucleotide polymorphisms in selected genes in inflammatory bowel disease. BioMed Research International. 2018;**2018**:6914346. DOI: 10.1155/2018/6914346

[15] Iida T, Onodera K, Nakase H. Role of autophagy in the pathogenesis of inflammatory bowel disease. World Journal of Gastroenterology.

2017;**23**(11):1944-1953. DOI: 10.3748/wjg.v23.i11.1944

[16] Boukercha A, Mesbah-Amroun H, Bouzidi A, Saoula H, Nakkemouche M, Roy M, et al. NOD2/CARD15 gene mutations in north Algerian patients with inflammatory bowel disease. World. Journal of Gastroenterology. 2015;**21**(25):7786-7794

[17] Sidiq T, Yoshihama S, Downs I. Kobayashi KSNod2: A critical regulator of ileal microbiota and Crohn's disease. Frontiers in Immunology. 2016;**20**(7):367

[18] Pranculienė G, Steponaitienė R, Skiecevičienė J, Kučinskienė R, Kiudelis G. Adamonis K, etal, associations between NOD2, IRGM and ORMDL3 polymorphisms and pediatric-onset inflammatory bowel disease in the Lithuanian population. Medicina (Kaunas, Lithuania). 2016;**52**(6):325-330. DOI: 10.1016/j.medici.2016.11.006

[19] Dai YE, Guan R, Song YT. The association of DLG5 polymorphisms with inflammatory bowel disease: A meta-analysis of 25 studies. European Review for Medical and Pharmacological Sciences. 2016;**20**:2324-2337

[20] Zhou Z, Zeng C, Guo C, Huang S, Huang C, Han Y, et al. A meta-analysis of P1371Q polymorphisms in DLG5 gene with reduced risk of Crohn's disease in European. International Journal of Clinical and Experimental Medicine. 2017;**10**(2):4107-4118

[21] Pieniążek M, Donizy P, Ziętek M, Szynglarewicz B, Matkowski R. Rola szlaków sygnalizacyjnych związanych z TGF-β w patogenezie przejścia nabłonkowo-mezenchymalnego (EMT) jako głównego elementu warunkującego progresję choroby nowotworowej. Postępy Higieny i Medycyny Doświadczalnejv. 2012;**66**:583-591

[22] Friedrichs F, Henckaerts L, Vermeire S, Kucharzik T, Seehafer T, Möller-Krull M, et al. The Crohn's disease susceptibility gene DLG5 as a member of the CARD interaction network. Journal of Molecular Medicine (Berlin, Germany). 2008;**86**(4):423-432

[23] Kubińska I, Pławski A, Czkwianianc E. Częstość polimorfizmów genu Nod2/Card15 w nieswoistych zapaleniach jelit u dzieci – materiał własny. Pediatr. Współcz. Gastroenterol. Hepatol. ZywienieDziecka. 2011;**13**(2):83-85

[24] Szeliga J, Sońdka Z, Jackowski M, Jarkiewicz-Tretyn J, Andrzej TA. Zarys immunopatogenezy choroby Leśniowskiego-Crohna ze szczególnym uwzględnieniem roli polimorfizmu genu NOD2/CARD15. Search Results. 2007;**14**(2):129-133

[25] Lin Z, Hegarty JP, Berg A, Wang Z, Kelly AA, Wang Y, et al. DLG5 P1371Q is associated with inflammatory bowel disease and complementary to R30Q in disease susceptibility. Swiss Medical Weekly. 2011;**8**:14

[26] Wang SL, Shao BZ, Zhao SB, Fang J, Gu L, Miao CY, et al. Impact of paneth cell autophagy on inflammatory bowel disease. Frontiers in Immunology. 2018;**9**:693. DOI: 10.3389/fimmu.2018.00693

[27] Nuij VJAA, Peppelenbosch MP, van der Woude CJ, Fuhler GM. Genetic polymorphism in ATG16L1 gene is associated with adalimumab use in inflammatory bowel disease. Journal of Translational Medicine. 2017;**15**(1):248. DOI: 10.1186/s12967-017-1355-9

[28] El-Khider F, McDonald C. Links of autophagy dysfunction to inflammatory bowel disease onset. Digestive Diseases. 2016;**34**(1-2):27-34. DOI: 10.1159/000442921

[29] Glas J, Seiderer J, Bues S, Stallhofer J, Fries C, Olszak T, et al.

IRGM variants and susceptibility to inflammatory bowel disease in the German population. PLoS One. 2013;**8**(1):e54338. DOI: 10.1371/journal.pone.0054338

[30] Zhao L, Xiao HT, Mu HX, Huang T, Lin ZS, Zhong LLD, et al. Magnolol, a natural polyphenol, attenuates dextran sulfate sodium-induced colitis in mice. Molecules. 2017;**22**(7):pii: E1218. DOI: 10.3390/molecules22071218

[31] Lamas B, Richard ML, Leducq V, Pham HP, Michel ML. Da costa G, etal, CARD9 impacts colitis by altering gut microbiota metabolism of tryptophan into aryl hydrocarbon receptor ligands. Nature Medicine. 2016 Jun;**22**(6):598-605. DOI: 10.1038/nm.4102

[32] Neavin DR, Liu D, Ray B, Weinshilboum RM. The role of the aryl hydrocarbon receptor (AHR) in immune and inflammatory diseases. International Journal of Molecular Sciences. 2018;**19**(12):pii: E3851. DOI: 10.3390/ijms19123851

[33] Boyd M, Thodberg M, Vitezic M, Bornholdt J, Vitting-Seerup K. Chen Y, etal, characterization of the enhancer and promoter landscape of inflammatory bowel disease from human colon biopsies. Nature Communications. 2018 Apr 25;**9**(1):1661. DOI: 10.1038/s41467-018-03766-z

[34] Tripathi K, Feuerstein JD. New developments in ulcerative colitis: latest evidence on management, treatment, and maintenance. Drugs Context. 2019;**8**:212572. DOI: 10.7573/dic.212572

[35] Brinar M, Cukovic-Cavka S, Bozina N, Ravic KG, Markos P, Ladic A, et al. MDR1 polymorphisms are associated with inflammatory bowel disease in a cohort of Croatian IBD patients. BMC Gastroenterology. 2013;**13**:57. DOI: 10.1186/1471-230X-13-57

[36] Roberts RL, Hollis-Moffatt JE, Gearry RB, Kennedy MA, Barclay ML, MerrimanTR. Confirmationofassociation of IRGM and NCF4 with ileal Crohn's disease in a population-based cohort. Genes and Immunity. 2008;**9**(6):561-565. DOI: 10.1038/gene.2008.49

[37] Manuc TE, Manuc MM, Diculescu MM. Recent insights into the molecular pathogenesis of Crohn's disease: A review of emerging therapeutic targets. Clinical and Experimental Gastroenterology. 2016;**9**:59-70

[38] Carrière J, Darfeuille-Michaud A, Nguyen HTT. Infectious etiopathogenesis of Crohn's disease. World Journal of Gastroenterology. 2014;**20**:12102-12117

[39] Ye BD, McGovern DP. Genetic variation in IBD: Progress, clues to pathogenesis and possible clinical utility. Expert Review of Clinical Immunology. 2016;**12**:1091-1107

[40] Freeman HJ. Natural history and long-term clinical course of Crohn's disease. World Journal of Gastroenterology. 2014;**20**:31-36

[41] Díaz Peña R, Valdés E, Cofré C, et al. Th17 response and autophagy - main pathways implicated in the development of inflammatory bowel disease by genome-wide association studies. Revista Española de Enfermedades Digestivas. 2015;**107**:560-566

Chapter 4

Single Nucleotide Polymorphisms (SNPs) in Plant Genetics and Breeding

Hande Morgil, Yusuf Can Gercek and Isil Tulum

Abstract

Recent advances in genome technology revealed various single nucleotide polymorphisms (SNPs), the most common form of DNA sequence variation between alleles, in several plant species. The discovery and application of SNPs increased our knowledge about genetic diversity and a better understanding on crop improvement. Natural breeding process which takes an agelong time during collecting, cultivating, and domestication has been accelerated by detecting dozens of SNPs on various species using advanced biotechnological techniques such as next-generation sequencing. This will result in the improvement of economically important traits. Therefore, we would like to focus on the discovery, current technologies, and applications of SNPs in breeding. The chapter covers the following topics: (1) introduction, (2) application of SNPs, (3) techniques to detect SNPs, (4) importance of SNPs for crop improvement, and (5) conclusion.

Keywords: SNPs, SNP identification, plant evolution, crop improvement

1. Introduction

Understanding the distribution and diversity of plant species is increasingly important to meet the demands of the growing population. Loss and deterioration have been observed in agricultural lands due to reasons such as salinization, environmental pollution, urban growth, temperature, and global climate change [1]. Prehistoric people were able to transform crops into crops that serve food for humanity by using traditional treatment techniques. These cultivated plants, when compared to their wild relatives, differed due to such characteristics that affected the plant breeders directly such as flowering time, sizes of the reproductive organs, and seed loss.

Significant improvements occurred in the productivity of agricultural products in the last century [2]. However, there are still areas in need of improvement. Today, there is still a great need for new genotypes in agricultural lands due to various social and cultural changes. Plant producers have to comply with the market needs, consumer demands, and growing agricultural problems. While much of the progress made so far has been achieved through classical improvement techniques, future prospects are under the control of biotechnology as a basic condition for achieving greater probability of success in product development [3]. In biotechnology, the study and use of DNA markers for plant breeding are encouraging for the future [4]. The use of DNA markers associated with crop yield is common in the development of various crops such as rice (*Oryza sativa*) [5], corn (*Zea mays*) [6], wheat (*Triticum aestivum*) [7], and tomatoes (*Lycopersicon esculentum*) [8].

If a single nucleotide change is detected by comparing the DNA of different living species, it is evaluated as there is a single nucleotide polymorphism. These changes in a single position are used as an effective genetic marker practically in both animal [9] and the plant [10, 11] species. Single nucleotide polymorphism (SNP) genotyping [12, 13] studies and the rapid progress in the development of genomic tools have led to the development of new powerful approaches in mapping complex features and identifying the causes.

In parallel with the increase in multidisciplinary studies and the development of technology, it is essential to use both traditional breeding techniques and new tools emerging in the field of molecular genetics [14]. In these tools, the two most used methods in terms of the low costs and high performance in obtaining data are microarrays and next-generation sequencing.

Since the end of the twentieth century, microarrays have been used in the first place to know the transcriptional activity of a biological sample [15]. Although other techniques have been previously used in gene expression studies such as northern blot or quantitative PCR, the ability to determine the level of less represented genes of a mixture facilitated the analysis of thousands of genes in the same reaction and increased sensitivity [16]. In the next-generation sequencing, the main goal is to parallelize DNA sequencing so that the molecules of thousands or millions of genetic materials could be read simultaneously. Regardless of the technique used, it identifies a large number of markers, allowing the development of high-density genetic maps [17]. This technology has been successfully used to detect SNPs of different genetically well-known species such as pine or corn [18, 19].

The wealth of data required to reveal evolutionary processes is based on highly efficient DNA sequencing. This technology enables nucleotide diversity studies related to a wide variety of species. The determination of the functionality of the genes of the wild species that have increased and continued in recent years and the presence of beneficial alleles for indirect plant breeding and yield improvement studies still make up an important topic for the future that is open for further improvement.

2. Applications of SNPs

Determining the DNA sequence variation in the genome is very important for plant genetics and breeding. Genetic variation can be analyzed using various molecular markers. The discovery of single nucleotide polymorphisms (SNPs), which underpin the difference between alleles, has been simplified and accelerated by recent advances in next- and third-generation sequencing technology and MALDI-TOF mass spectrophotometry compared to traditional methods [20]. Even creating machine learning models to select true SNPs directly from sequence data appears to be groundbreaking in this area [21].

The selection of SNPs enables the selection of desired lines in large-scale populations. The marker can be used to modulate the cultivation program for the determination of the relevant feature and improvement of the crop more economically using new-generation technologies than using traditional methods [22]. Today, plant breeding is dependent on SNPs and similar differences for fast and cost-effective analysis of germplasm and feature mapping. These differences improve the understanding of genetics that can change the strategy of developing new varieties.

Because the desired trait is under genetic control, phenotypic experiments can be attempted faster, and the breeder not only does the early trait selection but also can transmit the desired allele to a large number of populations [23].

As genomes of many species are fully sequenced, including human, *Arabidopsis*, and rice, the discovery of interest-specific sequence differences becomes easier [24]. These sequences enable screening of more than 1 million SNPs for each species. These polymorphisms can be used as simple genetic markers that can be identified around almost any gene. The usage of SNPs in detecting relationships between allelic forms of a gene and phenotypes, especially common diseases with multifactor genetics, high-resolution genetic map construction, linkage disequlibrium-based association mapping, genetic diagnostics, genetic diversity analysis, cultivar identification, and phylogenetic analysis, creates great potential for characterization of genetic resources [25]. SNPs are frequently found in the genome with at least one common (>20% allele frequency) SNP density per kilobase pair. It is mostly biallelic and therefore easy to analyze. More importantly, SNPs allow the combination of candidate gene approach and fusion-based fine mapping to identify the genes of interest [26].

The application of SNPs on genetic diversity is very important in terms of illuminating the relationships between varieties. This allows plant growers to improve crop plants and protect germplasm. Genetic diversity information can then be evaluated to identify new alleles in breeding programs. SNPs have been applied for several years to assess diversity in specific genes or genomic regions, and the results are estimated to extract phylogenetic relationships between species. However, the emergence of new and third-generation technologies allows the genome to assess SNP-based genetic diversity at scale and can be useful in conserving diversity in domesticated populations. Plant phylogenetic and evolutionary researches is traditionally based on sequence genes and hence the knowledge of SNPs [27]. Nuclear and chloroplast gene regions, which have been preserved for generations, are a rich source of phylogenetic information for evolutionary analysis in plants. The diversity and genotyping of the SNP sequence in these protected regions is used to explain a wide variety of phylogenetic and evolutionary relationships and inheritance extraction [28]. However, molecular phylogenetic studies only provide information about the distribution of populations, and contribution to agricultural applications is negligible compared to SNPs determined by transcriptome analyzes [29].

SNPs can also be used to discover new genes and their functions by affecting gene expression and transcriptional and translational promoter activities. Therefore, they may be responsible for phenotypic variations between individuals in improving agronomic features. It is also important to know the location of SNP in the genome, because if SNP is present in the coding region, it can greatly affect the activity and thermostability level of an enzyme or a similar product [30]. Sometimes it also depends on the substituted amino acid positions because some amino acid controls the activity of the expressed regions. Recent technological advances make it easier to identify various SNPs that can be used for product developments. It shows that SNPs in the functional parts of the gene can control the level of biotic and abiotic stress and improve the variety of abiotic and biotic stress tolerance crops by changing expressed region [31].

The integration of genomic technologies with traditional breeding can have a big impact in dealing with current and future environmental challenges more effectively [32]. In these conditions, germplasm in all plant species is imperative for rapid genetic gains in the productivity of these species using supportive approaches such as genetic and genomic sources.

3. Techniques to detect SNPs

The choice of the methods for SNP detection is diverse. The SNP detection technologies have been evolved with the discovery of new techniques on reporter systems, fluorescent probes, development of enzymatic assays, use of highly sensitive instruments, and mostly the accelerated high-throughput sequencing technology and bioinformatic tools. In the post-genomic era, the accuracy and sensitivity of the detection methods have increased with a cost-effective manner.

The basic idea behind SNP detection is whether identifying a novel polymorphism that is previously not defined or searching for an already-known polymorphism. The techniques for detection can be divided into two main groups: (i) in vitro and (ii) in silico techniques (**Figure 1**). In vitro techniques comprise of non-sequencing, sequencing, and re-sequencing methods.

3.1 In vitro techniques

3.1.1 Non-sequencing techniques

The firstly developed non-sequencing techniques are restriction digestion-based techniques such as restriction fragment length polymorphisms (RFLPs), cleaved amplified polymorphic sequences (CAPs), and derived cleaved amplified polymorphic sequences (dCAPs). These techniques mainly aim to create or disrupt a restriction enzyme recognition site [33]. Another group of non-sequencing technique is DNA conformation techniques which comprise denaturing gradient gel electrophoresis (DGGE), temperature gradient gel electrophoresis (TGGE), and single-strand conformation polymorphism (SSCP). The basis of these techniques is the separation of DNA fragments of the same length with different base composition on their three-dimensional conformation [34]. The chip-based methods are based on DNA hybridization like DNA microarrays and rely on the biochemical principle of nucleotide complementation. Affymetrix and Illumina SNP Chips use

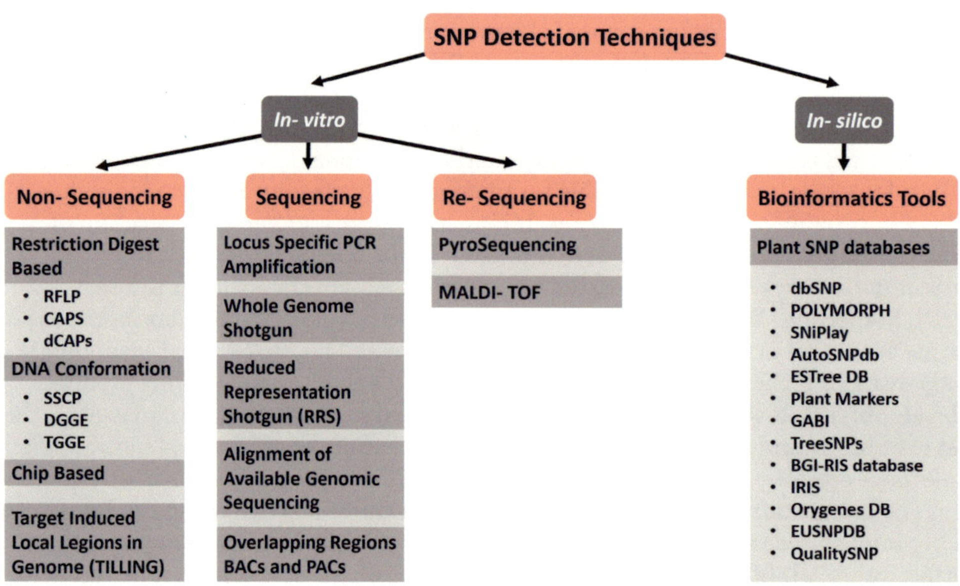

Figure 1.
Techniques to detect SNPs. In vitro techniques include non-sequencing, sequencing, and re-sequencing methods. In silico techniques basically includes bioinformatic tools with several output-/input-oriented algorithms.

the technology to hybridize fragmented single-stranded DNA to arrays containing thousands of nucleotide probe sequences that are designed to bind to a target DNA sequence [35]. Target-induced local lesions in genome (TILLING) is a reverse genetics approach that combines chemical mutagenesis with a sensitive mutation detection instrument called denaturing HPLC (DHPLC) [36]. The need of several optimization steps and "hundreds of bases"-long probes to detect only a small fraction of the region of interest made the non-sequencing methods very laborious and expensive. However, several newly developed approaches provide greater efficiencies. From all of these methodologies, direct DNA sequencing technologies are considered as the most used and benefited for SNP detection.

3.1.2 Sequencing techniques

One of the first designed sequencing-based techniques for SNP detection is locus-specific PCR amplification. In this approach, a large number of loci are targeted using locus-specific PCR primers and through conducting direct sequencing of genomic PCR products. Another sequencing-based technique is reduced representation shotgun (RRS). This method is based on the migration pattern of genomic segments of the same origin with the same size in gel electrophoresis [37]. Comparison in overlapped regions of bacterial artificial chromosome (BAC) or P1-derived artificial chromosome (PAC) clone regions is another sequencing-based approach for SNP discovery [38].

3.1.3 Re-sequencing techniques

Beside these techniques, there are re-sequencing approaches including matrix-assisted laser desorption ionization time-of-flight mass spectrometry (MALDI-TOF/MS) and pyrosequencing. MALDI-TOF/MS is based on differentiating genotypes by comparing the mass of DNA fragments after a single ddNTP primer extension reaction. This technique does not require labeling, and the detection depends on the mass of the ddNTP that is incorporated [39]. Pyrosequencing is a rapid re-sequencing approach in which the sequencing is performed by detecting the nucleotide incorporated by a DNA polymerase and monitored by a measure of pyrophosphate (PPi) release [40].

3.2 In silico techniques

As mentioned above, many experimental strategies are currently available for SNP detection. In vitro SNP detection methods are often composed of several laborious steps or require specialized instruments which makes the process high-cost and compound.

The developments in the sequencing technologies have resulted in decreasing cost along with rapid progress in next-generation sequencing (NGS) and related bioinformatic computing resources. These developments accelerated the whole-genome association studies (WGAS) and the identification of many new SNPs in model and non-model plants. In the post-genomic era, SNPs became the commonly used marker systems in many plants with several advantages such as stability, ease of use, considerably low mutation rates, and high-throughput genotyping [41]. NGS platforms generate a considerable amount of data in which results in the urge of alternative data storage methods and shorter processing time.

In silico methods are easy to apply to the SNPs that are occurring in known genomes or sequences of a species of interest. Bioinformatic research is constantly developing online and stand-alone tools, new software, and algorithms to analyze the SNPs. The recently developed open-source and freely available bioinformatic software have speed up the SNP detection and reduced the costs. The important point is the selection of the software, sequence platform, file requirement,

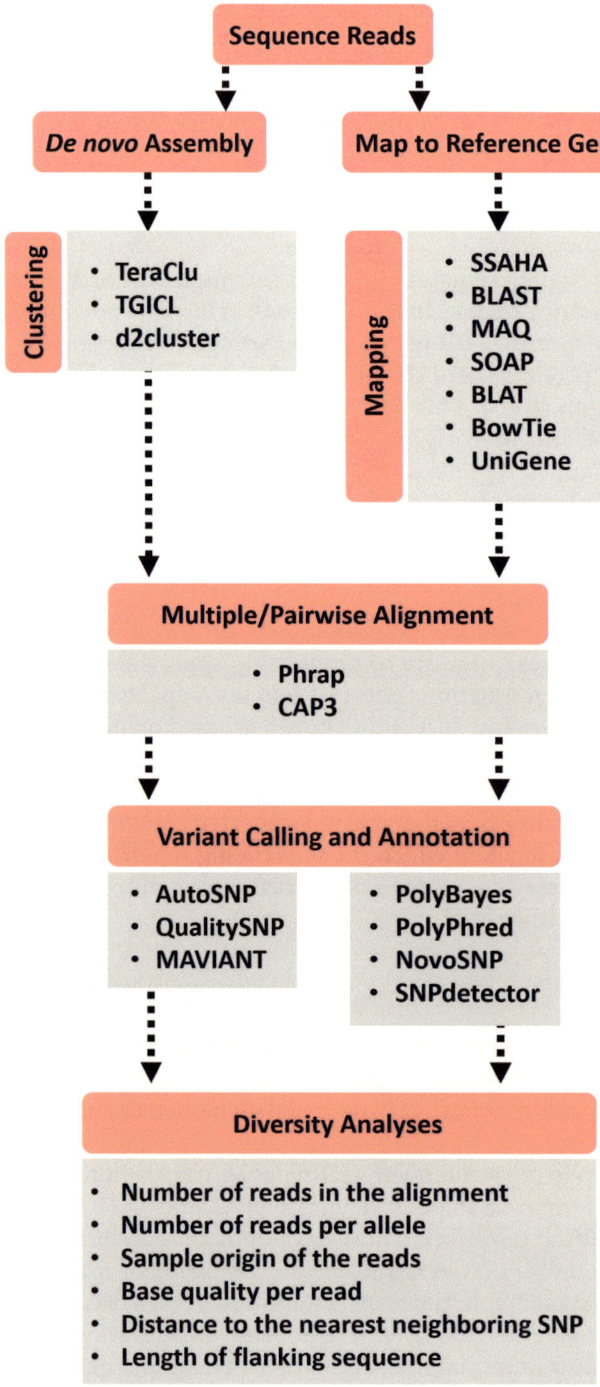

Figure 2.
A common workflow schema for in silico SNP mining. According to the input data type, the steps and the algorithms change. If the data set is de novo assembly output, clustering step is needed. If the data set is based on a reference mapped output, mapping step is required. In order to mine possible SNPs, after clustering and mapping steps, alignment, variant calling, annotation, and diversity analysis should be applied, respectively.

algorithmic background, operating systems, and organism of interest affect the choice of bioinformatic platform or pipeline to use. There are many databases and resources available today to describe SNPs in many plants.

The methods used for SNP mining will be quite similar for both database-derived and high-throughput sequencing-derived data. NGS technologies, Illumina GA/Solexa, SOLiDTM, Oxford Nanopore high-throughput sequencing, generate large amount of sequence data therefore many new SNPs. The method of choice may vary with different source data and varying approach. There are different analysis steps which apply to the two types of sequence data: reference sequence data where sequence data is acquired from species for which a reference sequence is accessible and de novo sequence data. In either case there are three main steps: (i) group the sequence reads according to their sequence similarities, and confirm identity of reads covering the same part of the genome or having the same transcript origin; (ii) align the reads; and (iii) scan for sequence variants (**Figure 2**).

If a reference sequence is available, the first step will be determining a homology search tool to map the new sequence reads to the reference. There are several tools for global or local mapping such as BLAST and SSAHA for whole-genome data. If the short reads are derived from Illumina, specially developed tools such as SOAP and MAQ are available. UniGene set is designed for mapping transcript data. The next step is to select a multiple or pairwise alignment tool to align the mapped reads to the reference sequence. Software tools like CAP3 and Phrap have been extensively used for this purpose.

In the case of de novo sequence data, an additional step called as clustering is needed to group the short sequence reads. TeraClu, TGICL, and d2cluster are the mostly used tools to fragmentate the input data and assemble them into individual contigs. After the clustering step, all nucleotides from individual reads at the identical position on the gene are aligned similarly using CAP3 and Phrap.

The final step is the SNP calling or validation. If the fragments are from a trace file or a base quality score, PolyBayes, PolyPhred, novoSNP, and SNPdetector are very well-known tools. If de novo SNP mining is performed, AutoSNP, QualitySNP, and MAVIANT can be used. There are several SNP mining tools or databases available specialized for plants such as dbSNP, ESTree DB, POLYMORPH, SNiPlay, AutoSNPdb, IRIS, etc. Although these tools are the frequently used, reliable and accurate tools, new tools, and platforms are being developed.

4. Importance of SNPs for crop improvement

Single nucleotide polymorphism (SNP) causes genetic diversity among individuals of the species and can occur at different frequencies in different species throughout the entire genome. SNPs can cause phenotypic diversity among individuals such as the color of different plants or fruits, fruit size, ripening, flowering time adaptation, crop quality, grain yield, or tolerance to various abiotic and biotic factors [42]. While SNPs can cause changes in amino acids in the exon of a gene, it can also be silent. In addition, it can occur in noncoding regions. SNPs can influence promoter activity for gene expression and finally produce a functional protein by transcription. Therefore, identifying functional SNPs in genes and determining their effects on the phenotype can lead to a better understanding of the effects on gene function for product development [43].

Conventional breeding and marker-assisted breeding are two approaches used to perform plant breeding [42, 44]. However, in plant breeding, publications on the application of molecular markers compared to conventional breeding have increased significantly over the past 15 years. Plant breeding forms and will continue to be the basis for increasing scientific efficiency in the field of food, feed, and industry. The reason why conventional breeding is increasingly preferred is that it requires hybridization between various parents and then selection over a long time (5–15 years) generation based on phenotypic selection to obtain the advanced product [45].

Rapid progress in sequence technologies, including SNP genotyping and genome sequencing, has given new and powerful approaches to mapping complex features and then identifying genes that cause this complexity. Although these methods are first applied in human genetics, their applications in plant genetics and product development are becoming popular [46]. With these new techniques, it is an important advantage to create experimental populations of germplasm collections and homozygous individuals in plants in a short time.

The most obvious advantages of SNP markers are that they are flexible and fast and provide data management convenience. For example, biallelic SNP markers are easy to combine data between groups and create large databases of this data because there are only two alleles for each location. This will also ensure the same allele detection on different genotyping platforms after appropriate quality assessment of these data. Using bioinformatic tools to transform SNP markers from different studies into the same DNA chain can contribute to improvement efforts [47]. With the help of a high-quality reference genome, the fusion sequence and SNPs also provide a stronger analysis of the entire SNP catalog for each species. As the most common type of DNA polymorphism, SNPs can also be specific at the genome-wide locus, which can reveal the selection of SNP variants at the target locus as well as informative marker sets for specific germplasm pools.

Due to the availability of technologies that provide validation and detection of SNPs, the development of SNP markers has become a routine process, especially in products with a reference genome. Appearance of whole-genome sequencing (GWAS) and de novo sequencing of unknown genomes has emerged. However, since 2006, it has been observed that SNPs have been used in publications derived from academic researches that have resulted in the development of crops such as water-tolerant rice, rust-resistant wheat varieties “Patwin,” and low phytic acid corn and, briefly, in order to correct the problems in agriculture. Although it does not normally disclose the details of reproductive methodologies to the public, it is known that SNP tokens have been applied in several articles published by companies such as Monsanto, Pioneer Hi Bred International, and Syngenta [48].

The effects on plant protein function and gene expression against a changing condition may result from SNPs occurring in coding regions and regulatory sequences, respectively. Therefore, SNPs have a great potential in genetic, reproductive, and economic importance [49].

Thus, the targeted product can be developed using only the data of the databanks before the fieldwork to efficiently cultivate a crop on logical and evolutionary studies. For example, in plant genetics, SNPs are widely used to identify the cis-regulatory variation within a species based on allele-specific analysis and to discover genes linked to complex genetic features by revealing its distribution, and it gives information about the adaptation of the species in that region. This situation also allows the investigation of the effects of changing conditions, especially by determining SNPs at the transcriptome level with RNA-seq technology. Using the RNA-seq data against two different conditions of the phenotype, you can create a SNP catalog and evaluate the effects on the protein sequence and which SNPs have a significant change in allele frequency. In addition, de novo and reference-based SNP discovery is carried out in many organisms, including many plants with little or no genetic information [50]. The availability of NGS provides a convenient approach to discover all SNPs and learn about genomic position and genotyping in one step. There are many advantages in performing SNP analysis using RNA-seq data. First, thousands of SNPs can be discovered, and expression levels of millions of functional genes with sequence variations can be observed simultaneously. Second, the location of variations in coding regions associated with biological and agronomic properties of plants can be identified, and phenotypes can be estimated by genotypes [51]. It also provides information for relevant studies such as gene characterization, gene expression measurement, and posttranslational process analysis. In addition, emerging technologies have allowed de novo scanning of SNPs computationally even in the absence of a reference genome sequence of any plant variety. Thus, the targeted product can be developed using only the data from data banks before the fieldwork to efficiently cultivate a crop [52]. The development and advancement of SNP technology are extensive for both evolutionary and molecular geneticists, plant breeders, and industry and will be valuable for us to understand and develop crop species.

5. Conclusion

In order to understand evolutionary and genetic relationships between/within species, elucidate traits of agronomic interest in crops, and clarify prone to diseases, SNPs are the first approach. Especially in plant genetic research and breeding, identifying the genetic loci that are responsible for trait variation is fundamental. With the advantages of stability, budget friendly improvements, and high-throughput assays, SNP has become increasingly important in crop genetic studies. The development of genotyping tools for model and non-model crops allows the detection of the variations, and it has been successfully applied in plant science for many years. The shift to the high-throughput genotyping assays and development of next-generation sequencing technologies accelerated the discovery of polymorphisms. However, the error-prone fashion of the NGS analysis tools is still a big concern which can lead to false-positive SNPs. There is a need for the development of a tool for extracting bulk of data, support for the data analyses, and intelligent decision on the accuracy. To fulfill this need, instead of using binary composition of nucleotides, machine learning approaches are being developed. Integrated SNP Mining and Utilization (ISMU) Pipeline is one of the first trials to develop a machine learning approach to SNP discovery. The integrated approach alongside the recent innovations will allow an increased knowledge and application of SNPs in the future.

Author details

Hande Morgil, Yusuf Can Gercek and Isil Tulum*
Department of Biology, Istanbul University, Istanbul, Turkey

*Address all correspondence to: iciltlm@gmail.com

References

[1] Backlund P, Janetos A, Schimel D. The effects of climate change on agriculture, land resources, water resources, and biodiversity in the United States. In: Synthesis and Assessment Product 4.3. Washington, DC: US Environmental Protection Agency, Climate Change Science Program; 2008. p. 240

[2] Bohra A et al. Genomics-assisted breeding in four major pulse crops of developing countries: Present status and prospects. Theoretical and Applied Genetics. 2014;**127**(6):1263-1291

[3] Lucht JM. Public acceptance of plant biotechnology and GM crops. Viruses. 2015;**7**(8):4254-4281

[4] Lateef DD et al. DNA marker technologies in plants and applications for crop improvements. Journal of Biosciences and Medicines. 2015;**3**(05):7

[5] Mackill DJ, Nguyen HT, Zhang J. Use of molecular markers in plant improvement programs for rainfed lowland rice. Field Crops Research. 1999;**64**(1-2):177-185

[6] Ortiz R. Molecular plant breeding. Crop Science. 2010;**50**(5):2196

[7] Suwarno WB et al. Genome-wide association analysis reveals new targets for carotenoid biofortification in maize. Theoretical and Applied Genetics. 2015;**128**(5):851-864

[8] Landjeva S, Korzun V, Börner A. Molecular markers: Actual and potential contributions to wheat genome characterization and breeding. Euphytica. 2007;**156**(3):271-296

[9] Illa-Berenguer E et al. Rapid and reliable identification of tomato fruit weight and locule number loci by QTL-seq. Theoretical and Applied Genetics. 2015;**128**(7):1329-1342

[10] Kim J-J et al. Development of SNP-based human identification system. International Journal of Legal Medicine. 2010;**124**(2):125-131

[11] Ganal MW et al. Large SNP arrays for genotyping in crop plants. Journal of Biosciences. 2012;**37**(5):821-828

[12] Ragousiss J. Genotyping technologies for genetic research. Annual Review of Genomics and Human Genetics. 2009;**10**:117-133

[13] Appleby N, Edwards D, Batley J. New technologies for ultra-high throughput genotyping in plants. Plant Genomics. Methods in Molecular Biology™ (Methods and Protocols). USA: Humana Press; 2009;**513**

[14] Perez-De-Castro M et al. Application of genomic tools in plant breeding. Current Genomics. 2012;**13**(3):179-195

[15] Slonim DK, Yanai I. Getting started in gene expression microarray analysis. PLoS Computational Biology. 2009;**5**:10

[16] Kerr MK, Martin M, Churchill GA. Analysis of variance for gene expression microarray data. Journal of Computational Biology. 2000;**7**(6):819-837

[17] Rasheed A et al. Crop breeding chips and genotyping platforms: Progress, challenges, and perspectives. Molecular Plant. 2017;**10**(8):1047-1064

[18] Eckert AJ et al. High-throughput genotyping and mapping of single nucleotide polymorphisms in loblolly pine (*Pinus taeda* L.). Tree Genetics & Genomes. 2009;**5**(1):225-234

[19] Yan J et al. High-throughput SNP genotyping with the GoldenGate assay in maize. Molecular Breeding. 2010;**25**(3):441-451

[20] Alonso-Blanco C, Andrade J, Becker C, Bemm F, Bergelson J, Borgwardt KM, et al. 1,135 genomes reveal the global pattern of polymorphism in *Arabidopsis thaliana*. Cell. 2016;**166**(2):481-491

[21] Bevan M, Walsh S. The Arabidopsis genome: A foundation for plant research. Genome Research. 2005;**15**(12):1632-1642

[22] Brachi B, Villoutreix R, Faure N, Hautekèete N, Piquot Y, Pauwels M, et al. Investigation of the geographical scale of adaptive phenological variation and its underlying genetics in *Arabidopsis thaliana*. Molecular Ecology. 2013;**22**(16):4222-4240

[23] Brennan AC, Méndez-Vigo B, Haddioui A, Martínez-Zapater JM, Picó FX, Alonso-Blanco C. The genetic structure of *Arabidopsis thaliana* in the south-western Mediterranean range reveals a shared history between North Africa and southern Europe. BMC Plant Biology. 2014;**14**(1):17

[24] Fournier Level A, Wilczek AM, Cooper MD, Roe JL, Anderson J, Eaton D, et al. Paths to selection on life history loci in different natural environments across the native range of *Arabidopsis thaliana*. Molecular Ecology. 2013;**22**(13):3552-3566

[25] Freudenthal JA, Ankenbrand MJ, Grimm DG, Korte A. GWAS-Flow: A GPU accelerated framework for efficient permutation based genome-wide association studies. BioRxiv. 2019;**1**:783100

[26] King G, Nienhuis J, Hussey C. Genetic similarity among ecotypes of *Arabidopsis thaliana* estimated by analysis of restriction fragment length polymorphisms. Theoretical and Applied Genetics. 1993;**86**(8):1028-1032

[27] Lasky JR, Des Marais DL, McKAY JK, Richards JH, Juenger TE, Keitt TH. Characterizing genomic variation of *Arabidopsis thaliana*: The roles of geography and climate. Molecular Ecology. 2012;**21**(22):5512-5529

[28] Nordborg M, Hu TT, Ishino Y, Jhaveri J, Toomajian C, Zheng H, et al. The pattern of polymorphism in *Arabidopsis thaliana*. PLoS Biology. 2005;**3**(7):1289-1299

[29] Purcell S, Neale B, Todd-Brown K, Thomas L, Ferreira MA, Bender D, et al. PLINK: A tool set for whole-genome association and population-based linkage analyses. The American Journal of Human Genetics. 2007;**81**(3):559-575

[30] Somerville C, Koornneef M. A fortunate choice: The history of Arabidopsis as a model plant. Nature Reviews. Genetics. 2002;**3**(11):883-889

[31] Xavier A, Muir WM, Rainey KM. Impact of imputation methods on the amount of genetic variation captured by a single-nucleotide polymorphism panel in soybeans. BMC Bioinformatics. 2016;**17**(1):55

[32] Yu C, Arcos-Burgos M, Baune BT, Arolt V, Dannlowski U, Wong ML, et al. Low-frequency and rare variants may contribute to elucidate the genetics of major depressive disorder. Translational Psychiatry. 2018;**8**(1):1-8

[33] Yu H, Xie W, Wang J, Xing Y, Xu C, Li X, et al. Gains in QTL detection using an ultra-high density SNP map based on population sequencing relative to traditional RFLP/SSR markers. PLoS One. 2011;**6**(3)

[34] Konstantinos KV, Panagiotis P, Antonios VT, Agelos P, Argiris NV. PCR–SSCP: A method for the molecular analysis of genetic diseases. Molecular Biotechnology. 2008;**38**(2):155-163

[35] LaFramboise T. Single nucleotide polymorphism arrays: A decade

of biological, computational and technological advances. Nucleic Acids Research. 2009;**37**(13):4181-4193

[36] McCallum CM, Comai L, Greene EA, Henikoff S. Targeting induced locallesions in genomes (TILLING) for plant functional genomics. Plant Physiology. 2000;**123**(2):439-442

[37] Altshuler D, Pollara VJ, Cowles CR, Van Etten WJ, Baldwin J, Linton L, et al. An SNP map of the human genome generated by reduced representation shotgun sequencing. Nature. 2000;**407**(6803):513-516

[38] Liu Z. Single nucleotide polymorphism (SNP). Aquaculture Genome Technologies. USA: Blackwell Publishing; 2007:59-72

[39] Bray MS, Boerwinkle E, Doris PA. High-throughput multiplex SNP genotyping with MALDI-TOF mass spectrometry: Practice, problems and promise. Human Mutation. 2001;**17**(4):296-304

[40] Storm N, Darnhofer-Patel B. MALDI-TOF mass spectrometry-based SNP genotyping. In: Single Nucleotide Polymorphisms. Totowa, NJ: Springer; 2003. pp. 241-262

[41] Ronaghi M. Pyrosequencing sheds light on DNA sequencing. Genome Research. 2001;**11**(1):3-11

[42] Huq MA et al. Identification of functional SNPs in genes and their effects on plant phenotypes. Journal of Plant Biotechnology. 2016;**43**(1):1-11

[43] Thomson MJ. High-throughput SNP genotyping to accelerate crop improvement. Plant Breeding and Biotechnology. 2014;**2**(3):195-212

[44] Kilian A et al. The fast and the cheap: SNP and DArT-based whole genome profiling for crop improvement. In: Proceedings of the International Congress in the Wake of the Double Helix: From the Green Revolution to the Gene Revolution. 2003. pp. 443-461

[45] Vera JC, Wheat CW, Fescemyer HW, Frilander MJ, Crawford DL, Hanski I, et al. Rapid transcriptome characterization for nonmodel organism using 454 pyrosequencing. Molecular Ecology. 2008;**17**:1636-1647

[46] Kwak M, Velasco D, Gepts P. Mapping homologous sequences for determinacy and photoperiod sensitivity in common bean (*Phaseolus vulgaris*). Journal of Heredity. 2008;**99**:283-291

[47] Shakira G, Azim A. Metagenomics and its application in rumen ecosystem: Potential biotechnological prospects. Pakistan Journal of Nutrition. 2009;**8**:1309-1315

[48] Varshney RK, Nayak SN, May GD, Jackson SA. Next generation sequencing technologies and their implications for crop genetics and breeding. Trends in Biotechnology. 2009;**27**:522-530

[49] Xu P, Wu X, Luo J, Wang B, Liu Y, Ehlers JD, et al. Partial sequencing of the bottle gourd genome reveals markers useful for phylogenetic analysis and breeding. BMC Genomics. 2011;**12**:467-477

[50] Duran C, Appleby N, Clark T, Wood D, Imelfort M, Batley J, et al. Auto SNPdb: An annotated single nucleotide polymorphism database for crop plants. Nucleic Acids Research. 2009;**37**:951-953

[51] McMullen MD, Kresovich S, Villeda HS, Bradbury P, Li H, Qi SQ. Genetic properties of the maize nested association mapping population. Science. 2009;**325**:737-740

[52] Imelfort M, Duran C, Batley J, Edwards D. Discovering genetic polymorphisms in next-generation sequencing data. Journal of Plant Biotechnology. 2009;**7**:312-317

Chapter 5

The Role of Genetic Polymorphisms in the Occupational Exposure

Pieranna Chiarella, Pasquale Capone and Renata Sisto

Abstract

In the last years, genetic polymorphisms have raised interest for their role on the environmental and occupational exposures. They not only are studied at population level to identify genetic diversity among ethnicities but have been recognized also as biomarkers of genetic susceptibility in many fields including medicine, health prevention, epidemiology and pharmacology. In the occupational context, the investigation of gene polymorphisms is part of the biomonitoring of workers exposed to occupational toxicants and carcinogens. However the majority of workers coming from foreign countries may be not familiar with the standard procedures used in the biomonitoring campaigns, which include human biosample harvesting for genetic, metabolic and genotoxic studies. Here we describe the importance of gene polymorphism association with dose and genotoxicity biomarkers and propose a statistical model predicting ethnic-specific susceptibilities based on the genotypes available in public databases when the access to blood genotyping test is not always feasible.

Keywords: biological monitoring, biomarker, biosample, environmental, ethnicity, gene polymorphism, occupational, susceptibility risk, worker

1. Introduction

The genetic variability is something common to all the living organisms and has important implications for the evolution and conservation of every species. It is widely known the differences in the phenotype among individuals are strictly dependent on two factors: the genotype, which is inherited from our ancestors, and the surrounding environmental exposure that contributes to shape the phenotype. The interindividual and intraindividual genetic differences make humans special and unique determining for each a single identity. Although genetics influences our physical appearance, behaviour, thoughts and habits, we recognize also the environment plays a crucial role in modifying many other parameters of our body. This depends on several factors: the country where we live, the ethnicity to which we belong to, the historical heritage, tradition and religion, the interaction with other people as well as the influence of the climate change on our life. If, on the one hand, our genetic heritage makes us unique, we acknowledge that classic genetics cannot explain the wide diversity of phenotypes within the population; nor classic genetics can explain the different phenotypes and disease susceptibility found in identical twins as well as in organisms obtained by cloning technology despite the DNA being exactly the same [1]. That means we cannot forget the strong influence of the surrounding environment on our genotype and on our physiological, physical and behavioral habits. Such influence, namely, epigenetics, means that the heritable changes in gene expression are not due to alteration in the DNA sequence but to some modifications occurring upon the DNA without changing the genetic code. That said, although we are aware the genetic variability is something peculiar to every human being, regardless of the inheritance of favorable or unfavorable genes, the transmission to the offspring will be modulated by epigenetics contributing to increase further the genetic variation in the population.

2. Variability among individuals: why it is important to study gene polymorphisms

Gene polymorphisms are the most common type of genetic variations in humans. They are present in the human population at frequency higher than 1% and differ from DNA mutations which are generally observed at extremely low frequency and in a restricted number of individuals. While gene polymorphisms are not necessarily associated to a specific disease, the gene mutation is generally known to cause a genetic disease. In humans the simplest type of polymorphism is the single nucleotide polymorphisms (SNPs), representing the most common type of nucleotide variation where a single base is substituted by another one (**Figure 1**). A SNP in the coding region of a gene may have four different effects on the resulting protein: (1) *synonymous substitution*, also known as silent mutation, causing no amino acid change in the protein, (2) *non-synonymous substitution* where a nucleotide mutation alters the amino acid sequence of a protein, (3) *missense substitution* consisting of an amino acid change with another and (4) *nonsense substitution* resulting in end of protein translation by a termination codon. About half of all the coding sequences of SNPs end up in non-synonymous codon changes. However SNPs may occur also in the regulatory region of the gene, affecting various properties of the protein. These SNPs may influence the protein in terms of quantity and quality, activity, processing and trafficking [2]. In the last 20 years, SNPs have raised a lot of

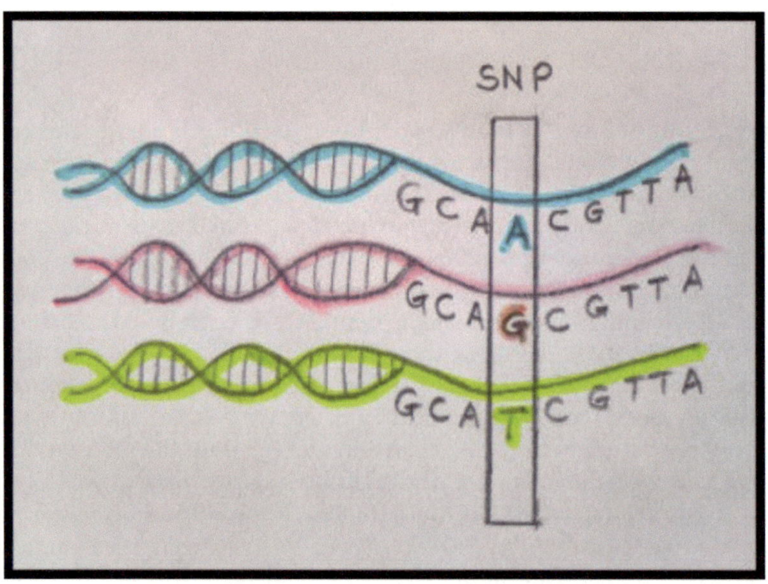

Figure 1.
Variation of single nucleotide in the human DNA coding sequence among individuals.

interest in many scientific fields related to public health and disease. They are also investigated in many scientific research areas, ranging from the human ethnicity study to the genetics of populations, personalized medicine, pathology, epidemiology, pharmacology, immunology and nutrition. More recently they have been considered relevant also for their role in the exposure science, a novel scientific branch linked to toxicology which characterizes and elucidates the contact of humans with dangerous chemical, physical and biological agents which represent a potential risk for the human health [3]. Actually the environmental exposure, in which also the occupational exposure is comprised, is acknowledged to play an important role in common chronic diseases, representing a major health concern in the economically developed countries. In this context the study of SNPs has a fundamental role to detect the human response to toxic and dangerous substances. Although the majority of SNPs of the human genome are of low prevalence [4], including the genes implicated in metabolism of environmental chemicals, these may substantially contribute to increase the population disease burden [5]. Since the exposure factors are numerous and several chronic diseases remain uncertain, it is fundamental to study the human genetic variation to understand the exposure-disease associations within the global population [6]. On the whole the genetic diversity associated to the variability of polymorphisms and to the genetic recombination is a valuable resource for humans and other living organisms. The interactions between the genetics of human beings and the surrounding environment reciprocally shape one with each other in order to reach an equilibrium. However such equilibrium might be perturbed by several exogenous factors such as the influence of natural selection, the global climate change, the re-emergence of extinct diseases and the admixing of different ethnicities due to massive migrations from one country to another. All these factors may contribute to change the variation of the gene polymorphism pool in the worldwide population. Nowadays the characterization of gene polymorphisms of the human population is carried out on individuals belonging to the same ethnicity so as to identify ethnic-specific gene/allele frequencies. This strategy should help geneticists to identify the genotype frequencies typical of members of a community sharing the same language, culture, religion, tradition, nationality, ancestry, nutrition, habits and lifestyle which influence the genetic background of the group [7]. For this reason the investigational studies of polymorphic genes refer more to the concept of ethnicity than to the race. The genetic characterization of separate ethnic groups provides useful information to evaluate the difference in the susceptibility risk of each cluster. Several papers have been published to report the typical genotype frequency of different gene polymorphisms in selected ethnicities [8–11]. However, due to the abundance of variation in gene polymorphisms, the characterization of the gene pool of a specific group of individuals is incomplete, and the genotype frequencies are known only for polymorphisms which have been investigated for their role or association to a specific susceptibility or disease. To our knowledge the commonest public databases collecting the gene polymorphisms available to the scientific community are the following: (1) the single nucleotide polymorphism database (dbSNP), a public archive for genetic variation hosted by the National Center for Biotechnology Information (NCBI) (https://www.ncbi.nlm.nih.gov/snp), and (2) the Ensembl project of genome databases for vertebrates and other eukaryotic species (http://grch37.ensembl.org/Homo_sapiens/Variation), which is the one we are using in the study of the human SNPs. These two archives represent a fundamental resource for our investigational studies on human genetic diversity when the laboratory genotyping is not feasible. In this chapter we describe some of our studies carried out during the biomonitoring campaigns of exposed workers where the biomarkers of dose, effect and susceptibility have been assessed in the occupational exposure. In addition we show also a statistical model we previously elaborated to identify ethnic-specific differences in the susceptibility risk to the typical exposure found in the workplace. In such model a statistical analysis has been done using the publicly available genotype frequency of four ethnic groups (Africans, East Asians, South Asians and Europeans) downloaded from the Ensembl project of genome databases.

3. Gene polymorphisms as susceptibility biomarkers in the occupational setting

It is widely known the exposure to dangerous substances and carcinogens is commonly associated to the individual capability of metabolizing such compounds which may vary between different individuals and among ethnicities, each characterized by its own specific genetic ancestry. In the occupational setting, the exposure risk is traditionally evaluated by the biological monitoring of workers manipulating hazardous agents. Common work-related substances are polycyclic aromatic hydrocarbons (PAH), a large class of organic compounds with carcinogenic properties (IARC group 1, 2B) used in the manufacture of chemicals, bitumen, and rubber and in shoe factories, while in fibreglass industries and in ship constructions, the most common dangerous substances are volatile organic compounds (VOCs) such as styrene (IARC group 2A), toluene (IARC group 3), xylene (IARC group 3), ethylbenzene (IARC group 2B) and benzene (IARC group I). The majority of these hazardous chemicals are highly toxic and carcinogenic to humans, and in each company, the officially approved occupational exposure limits (OELs) must be respected to ensure a safe environment for the workers' health. The procedure of workplace monitoring is generally standardized. It basically consists first of the environmental monitoring which measures the workers' airborne exposure to dangerous compounds and second of the biomonitoring which detects metabolites excreted in the biological specimens (urine, blood, saliva) and analyses the genotoxicity and gene polymorphisms in the subjects [12]. More specifically the biomonitoring allows to detect the following specific indicators: (i) the dose biomarkers, i.e. metabolites excreted in urine or in other bio-fluids; (ii) the early effect biomarkers, i.e. genotoxicity in peripheral blood lymphocytes and/or in buccal exfoliated cells; and (iii) the susceptibility biomarkers, i.e. the gene polymorphisms encoding for biotransformation enzymes during the exposure. This practice is carried out on exposed workers and nonexposed controls with the goal to assess the presence and quantify the potential health risks. While the dose biomarkers and the genotoxic damage may be immediately analyzed and quantified, the susceptibility biomarkers, being a qualitative parameter, are not quantifiable in terms of single polymorphism belonging to a subject. In such case the results obtained by the genetic analysis on groups of exposed workers have to be considered all together to quantify the relative susceptibility risk with respect to a control group. Based on our experience, the polymorphic genes of the worker population are identified following extraction of the genomic DNA of the subject to identify the genotype encoding the enzyme involved in the detoxification process. Once the worker genotype has been identified, it gives an important indication of the specific susceptibility to that substance by associating the genetic information with the dose and/or the early effect biomarker. In general the homozygous variant genotype (minor allele) is considered a risk allele with respect to the homozygous wild-type genotype (major allele) although there might be a few exceptions [13]. The workers exposed to potential hazardous substances are enrolled in the biomonitoring study only on a voluntary basis to allow the occupational health risk assessment. The results of the gene polymorphism assay together with the data gained by environmental and personal biomonitoring are analysed at the epidemiological level (1) to quantify the indoor exposure and the individual absorbed dose according to the company OELs for the specific hazardous agent, (2) to assess the potential genotoxic effect and (3) to evaluate the influence of the investigated polymorphic genes on the toxicant absorbed dose. Although workers make use of personal protection equipment (PPE), it is possible, in some cases, the high volatility of organic compounds might spread indoor, increasing the toxic substance threshold within the work environment. The finding of an association between the exposure to specific dangerous substances, the presence of cell genotoxicity and the variable functionality of gene polymorphisms are useful to identify specific or common susceptibilities in the exposed groups.

3.1 Identification of gene polymorphisms relevant to the occupational exposure

In our experience several biomonitoring studies have been promoted and carried out in industrial companies to assess the exposure risk of workers manipulating toxic and carcinogenic agents. Here we report the most recent results obtained during four different campaigns carried out in the last 6 years. In 2012, our research group analyzed the exposure of 315 workers to benzene in a petrochemical plant in Italy to evaluate the dose biomarkers S-phenylmercapturic acid (SPMA) and trans,trans-muconic acid (t,t-MA) in the worker urine samples and the susceptibility biomarkers in the blood specimens [14]. Since the GST enzymes may influence the metabolite excretion, the research project analyzed the association between metabolite excretion and contribution of the glutathione S transferase T1 (GST-T1) and M1 (GST-M1) polymorphisms to the detoxification. The results confirmed the modulating effect on the excretion of SPMA metabolite in urine by the genetic polymorphism of GST-T1 after exposure to low benzene doses. The same modulating effect was caused by the GST-M1 polymorphism but only at higher benzene doses, like those produced by cigarette smoking. The genotype of the 315 workers has been characterized to identify groups with the highest susceptibility; the workers' gene frequency of GST-T1 positive/null genotype was 0.78 vs. 0.22, while the frequency of GST-M1 positive/null was 0.47 vs. 0.53. Taking into account the genotype frequency of both enzymes, it looks that the GST-M1 polymorphism positive/null is less efficient in the detoxification process than GST-T1. A second study on benzene exposure has been carried out on 301 employees in the oil refinery. The effect of polymorphic genes GST-T1, GST-M1, glutathione S transferase A1 (GST-A1), epoxide hydrolase 1 (EHPX1), NAD(P)H quinone dehydrogenase 1 (NQO1), cytochrome P450 2E1 (CYP2E1), cytochrome P450 1A1 (CYP1A1*2A) and myeloperoxidase (MPO) involved in the detoxification of benzene has been analyzed. Here the dose biomarker was worked out as the ratio (R) between t,t-MA and S-PMA metabolites excreted in the urinary samples. The effect of smoking as confounding factor contributed to increase the relative production of S-PMA with respect to t,t-MA reducing the R value. This result was attributed to the higher levels of glutathione (GSH) in the red blood cells of smokers than in non-smokers. The analysis of susceptibility biomarkers showed a strong influence of GST-T1 positive polymorphism on the excretion of urinary S-PMA, reducing the conjugation rate of benzene epoxide with GSH in the GST-T1 null subjects. To a lesser extent, a similar effect was observed in individuals with GST-M1 null, GST-A1 and NQO1 mutant genotypes. It has been observed that in subjects with the double null GST-T1 and GST-M1 genotypes, an amplification of the t,t-MA biochemical pathway occurred with respect to the SPMA pathway [15]. However the activity of one GST is compensated by another in GST-M1 and GST-A1 defective subjects, but not in GST-T1 null genotypes, whose S-PMA average excretion is about 50% with respect to the positive genotypes for the same benzene exposure [16]. A further biomonitoring campaign has been conducted in two different manufacturing sites of central Italy on 30 styrene-exposed workers and 26 unexposed controls. In this work the authors investigated the effects of polymorphic genes CYP2E1, EPHX1, GST-T1 and GST-M1 on the urinary concentrations of the styrene metabolites, i.e. mandelic acid (MA) and phenylglyoxylic acid (PGA), and on the ratio between MA and PGA. Here the concentrations of urinary styrene and of airborne styrene have been determined. In the exposed workers, a lower excretion of PGA and MA metabolites was detected in subjects with cytochrome P450 2E1*5B (CYP2E1*5B) and cytochrome P450 2E1*6 (CYP2E1*6) heterozygous genotype with respect to the homozygous wild type indicating the influence of SNPs on the dose biomarkers. Furthermore a reduced value of metabolite ratio (MA + PGA/urinary styrene) was observed in exposed workers with the EPHX1 $Tyr^{113}His$ slow/mutant allele in comparison to those with the wild-type allele. The results indicate a reduced excretion of MA + PGA, evidenced also by other authors only in association with other genotypes. This study confirmed the variability in the excretion of urinary styrene metabolites, strictly related to the individual gene polymorphisms, can significantly impact on the biological monitoring of styrene exposure. In the CYP2E1*5B and CYP2E1*6 heterozygous genotypes as well as in the EPHX1 slow mutant genotypes, the average excretion of MA + PGA is, respectively, reduced 20 and 35% in comparison to the wild-type population [17].

3.2 Operative procedure and ethical use of workers' biosamples for occupational risk assessment

The availability of human biological samples is fundamental for the biomonitoring since it allows to estimate the exposure risk of the workers. The mostly used biosamples are whole blood with its separated fractions (plasma, serum, buffy coat, peripheral mononuclear cells, blood clot), urine, saliva, oral cell mucosa and cell components such as DNA and mRNA. In the occupational studies, biosamples are kindly donated from the workers agreeing to the biomonitoring project, provided that they give the informed consent. In Italy the biomonitoring procedure is sub-conditioned to the availability of the host manufacture company to agree the investigational study. The final purpose of the research has to be approved by the local health unit, by the research institute and, only in case of experimental clinical protocols, by the ethical committee. As volunteers the workers might join but not necessarily have to participate to the study related to the occupational health risk exposure, and they are not forced to undergo genetic screening. Workers participating to the programme agree by informed consent and are invited to fill a questionnaire to exclude all the potential confounding factors interfering with the analysis (drug assumption, alcohol consumption, smoking habit, chronic or acute diseases) before donating their biological samples. Those wishing to support the observational study are aware their specimens will be used only for the scientific purpose and will be collected, stored and used according to the ethical guidance of the Declaration of Helsinki [18]. The collection, storage and processing of the biosamples must be performed under strictly controlled procedures, in order to preserve their integrity and quality. In particular, the storage of genetic data collected in the workplace is fundamental since they contain sensitive health and non-health-related information about individuals which must be adequately protected in research as well as in clinical studies. This principle has been formalized in Europe on 27 April 2016 with the new General Data Protection Regulation (EU GDPR 2016/679), effective from 25 May 2018, which has entered into force and repealed the previous Directive 95/46/EC for personal data protection. The aim of the regulation is to promote and harmonize the personal data protection in the EU [19]. In the occupational setting, three types of biosamples are mainly requested to the workers, i.e. whole blood, urine and buccal cells. To perform genetic analysis on the biospecimen, the workers who agree to donate the sample must be informed of the purpose of the research project in all the aspects; they also should understand the utility, the scope and the limit of the analysis. Workers and their supervisors or representatives are informed on the modality, procedure and scheduling related to the donation of the biosamples. For instance, in the case of urine and buccal cells, workers can themselves self-collect their specimens provided that they are informed in advance on the day of collection. The collaborating institute ensures analysis of all the data, and for the genetic results, it ensures anonymity and confidentiality, un-disclosure in public databases, exclusivity and availability to medical staff of the company if required for internal use. Most importantly the genetic data are analysed as groups and not individually in order to avoid any misinterpretation or discrimination. As stated before, the information on the susceptibility risk is not relevant at the individual level, while it becomes significant once a large number of subjects belonging to the same ethnicity are available. The genetic analysis should be scientifically validated and must not involve any kind of discrimination for the individual.

3.3 Our method for gene polymorphism analysis

The workers' blood samples are harvested in tubes containing either heparin or K_2-EDTA from the medical staff of the company following workers' informed consent and according to the ethical guidelines of our research institute. All procedures performed in this study involving human participants [18] are in accordance with the ethical standards of our institutional committee and with the local health unit. Urine samples may be immediately frozen at −20°C after harvesting, and saliva and buccal cells may be stored at RT, while the blood samples may be stored up to 24 hours at a temperature between 4 and 10°C or immediately frozen for the genetic analysis. Blood genomic DNA is isolated by using a DNA blood kit, checked for the quality by agarose gel electrophoresis, quantified by a nanophotometer and stored at 4°C or −20°C. Although there are many novel and reliable techniques used to assess the gene polymorphisms such as Taqman assay, amplification refractory mutation system mass spectrometry (PCR-ARMS), confronting two-primer pair (CTPP-PCR), high-resolution melting and different types of mini-sequencing, our choice is oriented towards the traditional method based on polymerase chain reaction (PCR) followed by restriction fragment length polymorphism (RFLP) (**Figure 2**). We have tried also the fast and less expensive CTPP-PCR protocol developed previously in which the resulting genotype is obtained by a traditional PCR carried out with two couples of primers, avoiding to proceed for the enzymatic digestion [11]. However in our hands such protocol turned out

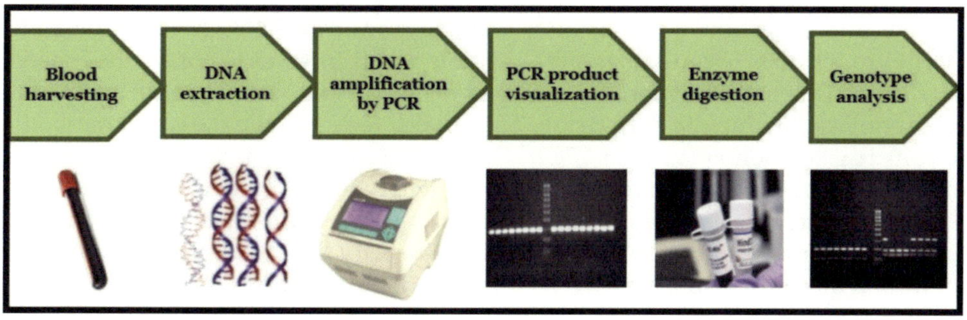

Figure 2.
Methodological procedure for gene polymorphism analysis by PCR-RFLP.

to be unreliable. In particular we applied this alternative method to detect two polymorphisms of one gene involved in response to oxidative stress and ototoxicity (NRF2 -617C/A and -653A/G), but the data were not completely satisfactory since CTPP-PCR produced contradictory results, particularly for the heterozygosis classification, requiring another orthogonal technique for confirming the data [20]. In the following section, we propose a list of the gene polymorphisms that we usually evaluate in the biological monitoring of the occupational exposure. They have been grouped on the basis of the enzyme function, i.e. detoxification, oxidative stress and DNA repair. The majority of them has been analyzed and reported in our previous published papers as biomarkers of susceptibility to the exposure of several organic compounds including styrene, toluene, ethylbenzene, benzene as well as biomarkers of genotoxic damage and of oxidative stress [14–17, 21]. **Table 1** shows a list of the analyzed susceptibility biomarkers together with the PCR-RFLP protocols which have been used by our group with some modifications.

3.4 Use of an alternative method to detect human gene polymorphisms without genotyping

In the context of occupational and environmental exposure, the role of biotransformation enzymes is to ensure efficient detoxification of endogenous and exogenous compounds by specific biochemical pathways. These modify the dangerous substances into inactive compounds which once excreted into urine will avoid metabolite accumulation and harm the human organism. Although the screening of individual gene polymorphisms by the molecular biology laboratory is the ideal procedure to assess the susceptibility of each individual participating to the study, the availability of workers to donate the biosample is fundamental to proceed with the genetic analysis. One difficulty may be represented by the lack of workers' consent to venipuncture or in general to the biosample harvesting, either because they are simply not used to this procedure or because the venipuncture is perceived as too invasive and painful technique or due to the worker fear and insecurity of the potential analysis result. However the gene polymorphism assessment has no diagnostic value in terms of predisposition to develop a particular disease. In our experience we noted that workers of mixed ethnicities are employed in many industrial companies, and in this context, it might be difficult, if not impossible, to collect particularly the blood samples in comparison to urine. This may depend on several factors: the poor knowledge of the language, the difficulty of communication and the difference in culture, habit, diet and belief among workers. To bypass such critical issue and achieve the ethnic-specific genotype information without making use of the laboratory analysis, we took advantage of a public and online available database (http://grch37.ensembl.org/Homo_sapiens/Variation) containing a provisional collection of the majority of genotype and allele frequencies of several ethnic groups. This resource is freely accessible and allowed us to obtain the genetic profile of different ethnicities which helped to predict and identify in silico specific susceptibilities within the population. This model, based on the statistical method of principal component analysis (PCA), has been designed to assess the relative risk of the homozygous variant and heterozygous genotype in four macro-groups, i.e. Africans, Eastern Asians, South Asians and Europeans, with respect to the worldwide population [34]. It has been conceived to identify the critical susceptibilities in the polymorphisms of genes involved in three main functional biochemical pathways, i.e. detoxification, oxidative stress and repair of damaged DNA, following exposure to the hazardous compounds. The SNPs have been selected on the basis of the exposure to toxic and carcinogenic substances commonly found in manufacturing factories and shipyards. Below we list the gene polymorphisms

SNPs	rs number	Primer sequences	Annealing temperature (°C)	Restriction enzyme	Restriction pattern (bp)	References
Detoxification						
GST-T1	17856199	F: 5′ -TTC CTT ACT GGT CCT CAC ATC TC-3′ R: 5′ -TCA CCG GAT CAT GGC CAG CA-3′	62	None	None	Teixeira et al. [22]
GST-M1	366631	F: 5′-GAA CTC CCT GAA AAG CTA AAG C-3′ R: 5′-GTT GGG CTC AAA TAT ACG GTG G-3′	62	None	None	
GST-P1	1695	F: 5′-ACC CCA GGG CTC TAT GGG AA-3′ R: 5′-TGA GGG CAC AAG AAG CCC CT-3′	62	BsmAI	Wt: 176 Het: 176, 91, 85 Mut: 91, 85	
GST-A1	3957357	F: 5′-GCA TCA GCT TGC CCT TCA-3′ R: 5′-AAA CGC TGT CAC CGT CCTG-3′	64	EarI	Wt: 400 Het: 400, 308, 92 Mut: 308, 92	Ping et al. [23]
CYP1A1*2A	4646903	F: 5′-CAGTGAAGAGGTGTAGCCGCT3′ R: 5′-TAGGAGTCTTGTCTCATGCCT3′	65	MspI	Wt: 340 Het: 340, 200, 140 Mut: 200, 140	Nie et al. [24]
CYP2E1*5B	3813867	F: 5′-CCA GTC GAG TCT ACA TTG TCA-3′ R: 5′-TTC ATT CTG TCT TCT AAC TGG-3′	55	RsaI	Wt: 360, 50 Het: 410, 360, 50 Mut: 410	Le Marchand et al. [25]
CYP2E1*intron6	6413432	F: 5′-TCG TCA GTT CCT GAA AGC AGG-3′ R: 5′-GAG CTC TGA TGC AAG TAT CGC A-3′	62	DraI	Wt: 572, 302, 121 Het: 874, 572, 302, 121, Mut: 874, 121	Liu et al. [26]
EPHX1 Ex_3	1051740	F: 5′-GAT CGA TAA GTT CCG TTT CAC C-3′ R: 5′-ATC CTT AGT CTT GAA GTG AGG AT-3′	52.6	EcoRV	Wt: 160 Het: 160, 140, 20 Mut: 140, 20	Erkisi et al. [27]
EPHX1 Ex_4	2234922	F: 5′-GGG GTA CCA GAG CCT GAC CGT-3′ R: 5′-AAC ACC GGG CCC ACC CTT GGC-3′	58	RsaI	Wt: 295, 62 Het: 295, 174, 62 Mut: 174, 121, 62	Hassett et al. [28]
MPO	2333227	F: 5′-CGG TAT AGG CAC ACA ATG GTG AG-3′ R: 5′-GCA ATG GTT CAA GCG ATT CTT C 3’	56	AciI	Wt: 168, 121, 61 Het: 289, 168, 121, 61 Mut: 289, 61	Cascorbi et al. [29]

SNPs	rs number	Primer sequences	Annealing temperature (°C)	Restriction enzyme	Restriction pattern (bp)	References
Oxidative stress						
NRF2 – 617C/A	6721961	F1 5′- CCC TGA TTT GGA GTT GCA GAA CC-3′ R2 5′- CTC CGT TTG CCT TTG ACG AC-3′	62	NgoMIV	Wt: 191, 91 Het: 281, 191, 91 Mut: 282	Chiarella et al. [20]
NRF2 – 653A/G	35652124	F1 5′-CTT TTA TCT CAC TTT ACC GCC CGA G-3’ R2 5’-GGG GTT CCC GTT TTT CTC CC-3′	62	BseRI	Wt: 180, 138 Het: 318, 280,180, Mut: 318	
NQO1	1800566	F: 5′-TCC TCA GAG TGG CAT TCT GC-3′ R: 5′-TCT CCT CAT CCT GTA CCT CT-3′	65	HinfI	Wt: 195 Het: 195, 151, Mut: 151	Chen et al. [30]
HO-1	2071746	5′-GTT CCT GAT GTT GCC CAC CAA GC-3′ 5′-CTG CAG GCT CTG GGT GTG ATT TTG-3′	60	HindIII	Wt: 131 Het: 20, 131 Mut: 20	Song et al. [31]
DNA repair						
XRCC1 399 G/A	25487	F: 5′-TTG TGC TTT CTC TGT GTC CA-3′ R: 5′-TCC TCC AGC CTT TTC TGA TA-3′	61	MspI	Wt: 374, 221 Het: 615, 374, 221 Mut: 615	Kowalski et al. [32]
XRCC1 194	1799782	F: 5′-GCC CCG TCC CAG GTA-3′ R: 5’-AGC CCC AAG ACC CTT TCA TC-3’	61	MspI	Wt: 292, 174 Het: 313, 292, 174 Mut: 313, 174	
hOGG1 326	1,052,133	F: 5′-GGA AGG TGC TTG GGG AAT-3′ R: 5′-ACT GTC ACT AGT CTC ACC AG-3’	58	Fnu4HI	Wt: 200 Het: 200, 100 Mut: 100	Le Marchand et al. [33]

Wt, Homozygous wild type; Het, heterozygous; Mut, homozygous mutant.

Table 1.
List of susceptibility biomarkers analysed in our biomonitoring campaigns.

reported in **Table 1** and commonly assessed in the laboratory genotyping during the biomonitoring campaigns that in our predictive model we integrated with other relevant polymorphic genes [34].

1. Detoxification pathway genes: Glutathione S transferase (GST-A1) rs3957357, (GST-M1) rs366631, (GST-T1) rs17856199, (GST-P1) rs1695, epoxide hydrolase 1 (EPHX1 Ex_3) rs1051740, (EPHX1 Ex_4) rs2234922, cytochrome P450 1A1 (CYP1A1_2A) rs4646903, cytochrome P450 2E1 (CYP2E1*6) rs6413432, (CYP2E1*5B) rs3813867, myeloperoxidase (MPO) rs2333227.

2. Oxidative stress genes: Nuclear factor (erythroid-derived 2)-like 2 (NRF2) rs6721961, NRF2 rs35652124, heme oxygenase (HO-1) rs2071746, NAD(P)H quinone dehydrogenase 1 (NQO1) rs1800566.

3. DNA repair pathway genes: X-ray repair cross-complementing 1 (XRCC1) rs25487, X-ray repair cross-complementing 3 (XRCC3) rs1799782, 8-oxoguanine glycosylase (hOGG1) rs1052133.

The model provides the relative risk (RR) for each ethnic group. RR has been calculated as the ratio between the variations of the gene frequency of the specific ethnic group with respect to the variation of the gene frequency of the worldwide population. If the variation of the gene frequency is >1, it means the susceptibility risk is higher in the ethnic group than in the general population. The most disadvantageous condition, unless specified, is generally associated with the frequency of the homozygous variant, namely, the mutant genotype, although in very few exceptions it might associate to the homozygous wild-type genotype. The details of the rationale, method and elaboration of the susceptibility relative risk of the model are available in our previous paper [34]. Briefly, the predictive model allows to identify (1) ethnicity similarity in the susceptibility risk, (2) correlation of the ethnicity with specific metabolic genes and (3) estimation of the RR indicator in the four ethnic macro-populations. In **Figure 3** we report a quantification of the RR for all the four ethnic groups which has been worked out for the three gene polymorphism clusters (i.e. detoxification, oxidative stress and DNA repair). As seen in the graph, the

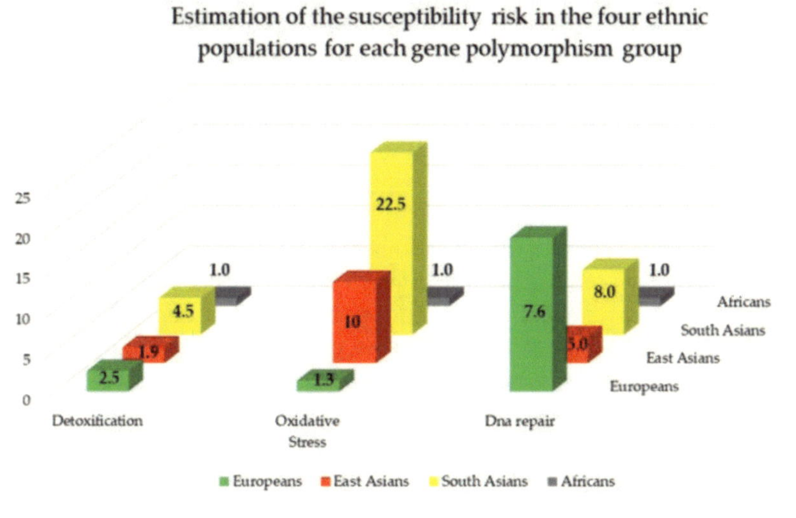

Figure 3.
Calculation of the indicator risk in the four ethnic populations.

minimum risk for the three categories of gene polymorphisms is observed in the case of Africans, while South Asians are associated to the highest risk for detoxification and oxidative stress; Europeans show the highest risk in the DNA repair; and East Asians show a high risk in the oxidative stress. According to the following results, it seems that South Asians are associated with a cumulative highest susceptibility risk in comparison to the other populations, while Africans are associated to the lowest risk. The model cited here may represent a useful tool to predict the susceptibility risk associated to the occupational exposure and a potential alternative substituting the genotype screening of workers. However, it is still provisional, and it could be improved considering other ethnicities and including in the analysis a higher number of polymorphic genes involved in the biotransformation of the toxic and carcinogenic substances found in the workplace.

4. Conclusions

The recent and massive migration of populations of various ethnicities in the European countries and the global climate changes not only are affecting the human social life and behaviors but represent also a serious health and safety concern for the population. Any individual response to the environmental and occupational exposure is dependent on different factors; one of the most important and obvious is related to the personal genetic background characterizing different population groups. However many other exogenous factors such as the individual lifestyle, the smoking habit, the use of drugs, the type of diet and the ubiquitous presence of toxicants are factors affecting the individual genetic heritage. A novel and effective approach to the management of the public health risk is urgently needed. Although the genetic information is correctly used in the occupational risk assessment models, various ethical and social issues may arise when dealing with gene polymorphisms at workplace, particularly when the labour force is heterogeneous. The possible reluctance of immigrants and of local workers to give the consent to the biosample donation, the expenses sustained by the laboratory for the analysis as well as the necessity of approvals by the health unit and the manufacturing company to allow the investigational study do not facilitate the success of the biomonitoring campaign which, if not mandatory as the health surveillance, is still important to assess and quantify the exposure to hazardous substances and the susceptibility risk at workplace. Nonetheless the worker misinterpretation or the miscommunication of genetic susceptibility and vulnerability concepts might be misunderstood and considered as personal weakness or inability to perform a specific job task. This erroneous interpretation of susceptibility should be transferred to the workers in a clear and correct form so as they know the individual variability, regardless of the difference in genetic heritage, is not a negative aspect but should be conceived as a personal trait. The role of genotyping in the occupational exposure, no matter if it is carried out in a laboratory or by a statistical analysis, is to define a susceptibility risk for the investigated ethnic group. This information will be useful to take into account the difference between ethnicities so as to verify the company OELs are safe or need to be adjusted taking into account different susceptibilities. In the absence of blood sample or consent from the worker to donation, the availability of a statistical predictive model, based on the genotype publicly available on web databases, should be necessarily regarded as useful indicator of the probable subject's genotype of the ethnic group to which the individual belongs to. Even though the access to genotyping is not possible, a certain number of advantages might be achieved: reduction of the laboratory costs for the research institute, no need of informed consent from workers and no need of trained staff and laboratory equipment for blood collection and therefore no venipuncture, which means no harm to the worker. The predictive model mentioned here may represent a potential but also amendable alternative to the laboratory genotyping of workers and might involve the study of other ethnic groups. However keeping updated these databases will be useful not only to better characterize all the ethnic groups' genotypes but also to manage the novel susceptibility risks that might compromise the individual health protection and safety in the workplace [35].

Acknowledgements

The authors thank all the colleagues of our institute with whom we collaborated to the biomonitoring investigational studies. No fundings have been used to write this chapter.

Conflict of interests

The authors declare no conflict of interest.

Author details

Pieranna Chiarella*, Pasquale Capone and Renata Sisto*
Department of Occupational and Environmental Medicine, Epidemiology and Hygiene, INAIL–Italian National Workers', Compensation Authority, Research Center of Monteporzio Catone, Rome, Italy

*Address all correspondence to: p.chiarella@inail.it and r.sisto@inail.it

References

[1] Esteller M. Epigenetics in cancer. The New England Journal of Medicine. 2008;**358**:1148-1159. DOI: 10.1056/NEJMra072067

[2] Buckland PR. The importance and identification of regulatory polymorphisms and their mechanisms of action. Biochimica et Biophysica Acta. 2006;**1762**:17-28. DOI: 10.1016/j.bbadis.2005.10.004

[3] Lioy P, Lebret E, Spengler J, Brauer M, Buckley T, Freeman N, et al. Defining exposure science. Journal of Exposure Analysis and Environmental Epidemiology. 2005;**15**(6):463. DOI: 10.1038/sj.jea.7500463

[4] Vineis P, Ahsan H, Parker M. Genetic screening and occupational and environmental exposures. Occupational and Environmental Medicine. 2005;**62**:657-662. DOI: 10.1136/oem.2004.019190

[5] Vineis P, Schulte P, McMichael AJ. Misconceptions about the use of genetic tests in populations. Lancet. 2001;**357**:709-712. DOI: 10.1016/S0140-6736(00)04136-2

[6] Wild CP. Complementing the genome with an "exposome": The outstanding challenge of environmental exposure measurement in molecular epidemiology. Cancer Epidemiology, Biomarkers and Prevention. 2005;**14**:1847-1850. DOI: 10.1158/1055-9965.EPI-05-0456

[7] Morin MM, Pickle LW, Mason TJ. Geographic patterns of ethnic groups in the United States. American Journal of Public Health. 1984;**74**:133-139

[8] Kasthurinaidu SP, Ramasamy T, Ayyavoo J, Dave DK, Adroja DA. GST M1-T1 null allele frequency patterns in geographically assorted human populations: A phylogenetic approach. PLoS One. 2015;**10**(4):e0118660. DOI: 10.1371/journal.pone.0118660

[9] Zhou HH, Liu ZQ. Ethnic differences in drug metabolism. Clinical Chemistry and Laboratory Medicine. 2000;**38**: 899-903. DOI: 10.1515/CCLM.2000.131

[10] McGraw J, Waller D. Cytochrome P450 variations in different ethnic populations. Expert Opinion on Drug Metabolism and Toxicology. 2012;**8**: 371-382. DOI: 10.1517/17425255.2012.657626

[11] Hamajima N, Saito T, Matsuo K, Kozaki K, Takahashi T, Tajima K. Polymerase chain reaction with confronting two-pair primers for polymorphism genotyping. Japanese Journal of Cancer Research. 2000;**91**:865-868

[12] Ladeira C, Viegas S. Human biomonitoring—An overview on biomarkers and their application in occupational and environmental health. Biomonitoring. 2016;**3**:15-24. DOI: 10.1289/ehp.6065

[13] Kido T, Sikora-Wohlfeld W, Kawashima M, Kikuchi S, Kamatani N, Patwardhan A, et al. Are minor alleles more likely to be risk alleles. BMC Medical Genomics. 2018;**11**(1):3. DOI: 10.1186/s12920-018-0322-5

[14] Mansi A, Bruni R, Capone P, Paci E, Pigini D, Simeoni C, et al. Low occupational exposure to benzene in a petrochemical plant: Modulating effect of genetic polymorphisms and smoking habit on the urinary t,t-MA/SPMA ratio. Toxicology Letters. 2012;**213**:57-62

[15] Pavanello S, Clonfero E. Biological indicators of genotoxic risk and metabolic polymorphisms. Mutation Research. 2000;**463**:285-308

[16] Carbonari D, Proietto A, Fioretti M, Tranfo G, Paci E, Papacchini M, et al.

Influence of genetic polymorphism on t,t-MA/S-PMA ratio in 301 benzene exposed subjects. Toxicology Letters. 2014;**231**:205-212. DOI: 10.1016/j.toxlet.2014.06.029

[17] Carbonari D, Mansi A, Proietto AR, Paci E, Bonanni RC, Gherardi M, et al. Influence of genetic polymorphisms of styrene-metabolizing enzymes on the levels of urinary biomarkers of styrene exposure. Toxicology Letters. 2015;**233**:156-162

[18] World Medical Association. World Medical Association Declaration of Helsinki: Ethical principles for medical research involving human subjects. Journal of the American Medical Association. 2013;**310**:2191-2194. DOI: 10.1001/jama.2013.281053

[19] Shabani M, Borry P. Rules for processing genetic data for research purposes in view of the new EU General Data Protection Regulation. European Journal of Human Genetics. 2018;**26**:149-156. DOI: 10.1038/s41431-017-0045-7

[20] Chiarella P, Sisto R, de Marco A. Confronting two biomolecular techniques to detect NRF2 gene polymorphism biomarkers. Future Science OA. 2018;**5**(2):FSO361. DOI: 10.4155/fsoa-2018-0075

[21] Sisto R, Capone P, Cerini L, Sanjust F, Paci E, et al. Circulating microRNAs as potential biomarkers of occupational exposure to low dose organic solvents. Toxicology Reports. 2019;**6**:126-135. DOI: 10.1016/j.toxrep.2019.01.001

[22] Teixeira JP, Gaspar J, Silva S, Torres J, Silva SN, Azevedo MC, et al. Occupational exposure to styrene: Modulation of cytogenetic damage and levels of urinary metabolites of styrene by polymorphisms in genes CYP2E1, EPHX1, GSTM1, GSTT1 and GSTP1. Toxicology. 2004;**195**(2-3):231-242. DOI: 10.1016/j.tox.2003.10.010

[23] Ping J, Wang H, Huang M, Liu ZS. Genetic analysis of glutathione S-transferase A1 polymorphism in the Chinese population and the influence of genotype on enzymatic properties. Toxicological Sciences. 2006;**89**(2):438-443. DOI: 10.1093/toxsci/kfj037

[24] Nie Q, Yang XN, An SJ, Zhang XC, Yang JJ, Zhong WZ, et al. CYP1A1*2A polymorphism as a predictor of clinical outcome in advanced lung cancer patients treated with EGFR-TKI and its combined effects with EGFR intron 1 (CA)n polymorphism. European Journal of Cancer. 2011;**47**(13):1962-1970. DOI: 10.1016/j.ejca.2011.04.018

[25] Le Marchand L, Wilkinson GR, Wilkens LR. Genetic and dietary predictors of CYP2E1 activity: A phenotyping study in Hawaii Japanese using chlorzoxazone. Cancer Epidemiology, Biomarkers and Prevention. 1999;**8**(6):495-500

[26] Liu R, Yin LH, Pu YP. Association of combined CYP2E 1 gene polymorphism with the risk for esophageal squamous cell carcinoma in Huai'an population China. Chinese Medical Journal. 2007;**120**(20):1797-1802

[27] Erkisi Z, Yaylim-Eraltan I, Turna A, Görmüs U, Camlica H, Isbir T. Polymorphisms in the microsomal epoxide hydrolase gene: Role in lung cancer susceptibility and prognosis. Tumori. 2010;**96**(5):756-763. DOI: 10.1177/030089161009600519

[28] Hassett C, Aicher L, Sidhu JS, Omiecinski CJ. Human microsomal epoxide hydrolase: Genetic polymorphism and functional expression in vitro of amino acid variants. Human Molecular Genetics. 1994;**3**(3):421-428

[29] Cascorbi I, Henning S, Brockmöller J, Gephart J, Meisel C, Müller JM, et al. Substantially reduced risk of cancer of the aerodigestive tract in subjects with variant- 463A of the

myeloperoxidase gene. Cancer Research. 2000;**60**(3):644-649

[30] Chen H, Lum A, Seifried A, Wilkens LR, Le Marchand L. Association of the NAD(P)H: Quinone oxidoreductase ^{609}→C T polymorphism with a decreased lung cancer risk. Cancer Research. 1999;**59**(13):3045-3048

[31] Song P, Li K, Liu L, Wang X, Jian Z, Zhang W, et al. Genetic polymorphism of the Nrf2 promoter region is associated with vitiligo risk in Han Chinese populations. Journal of Cellular and Molecular Medicine. 2016;**20**(10):1840-1850. DOI: 10.1111/jcmm.12874

[32] Kowalski M, Przybylowska K, Rusin P, Olszewski J, Morawiec-Sztandera A, Bielecka-Kowalska A, et al. Genetic polymorphisms in DNA base excision repair gene XRCC1 and the risk of squamous cell carcinoma of the head and neck. Journal of Experimental and Clinical Cancer Research. 2009;**28**:37. DOI: 10.1186/1756-9966-28-37

[33] Le Marchand L, Donlon T, Lum-Jones A, Seifried A, Wilkens LR. Association of the hOGG1 Ser326Cys polymorphism with lung cancer risk. Cancer Epidemiology, Biomarkers and Prevention. 2002;**11**(4):409-412

[34] Chiarella P, Capone P, Carbonari D, Sisto R. A predictive model assessing the genetic susceptibility risk at workplace. International Journal of Environmental Research and Public Health. 2019;**16**:2012. DOI: 10.3390/ijerph16112012

[35] Kelada SN, Eaton DL, Wang SS, Rothman NR, Khoury MJ. The role of genetic polymorphisms in environmental health. Environmental Health Perspectives. 2003;**111**:1055-1064. DOI: 10.1289/ehp.6065

Chapter 6

The Protein Tyrosine Phosphatase Non-Receptor Type 22 (PTPN22) Gene Polymorphism and Susceptibility to Autoimmune Diseases

Ghaleb Bin Huraib, Fahad Al Harthi, Misbahul Arfin and Abdulrahman Al-Asmari

Abstract

The protein tyrosine phosphatase non-receptor type 22 (PTPN22) gene located on chromosomes 1p 13.3–13 encodes a lymphoid-specific tyrosine phosphatase (Lyp) which is involved in autoimmunity by preventing spontaneous T-cell activation and T-cell development and inactivating T-cell receptor-associated kinases and their substrates. Several single nucleotide polymorphisms (SNPs) have been identified in PTPN22, but only one PTPN22 C1858T has been intensively studied in relation to autoimmune diseases. The PTPN22 C1858T functional polymorphism is a strong non-HLA risk factor for several autoimmune diseases and considered to play an important role in etiology of diseases due to significant production of autoantibodies. However, available literature on PTPN22 C1858T polymorphism and autoimmune diseases shows inconsistencies and ethnic variations. Therefore, further genetic studies on patients suffering from various autoimmune diseases from different ethnicities and PTPN22 gene polymorphisms are expected to help better understand the pathogenesis and will contribute to the development of more targeted therapies and biomarkers.

Keywords: PTPN22, genetic, polymorphism, autoimmune diseases

1. Introduction

Genetic polymorphisms are variations in DNA found in 1% or more of the population which may alter the structure and function of protein through a single nucleotide base substitution in a gene's coding region. It may alter the gene expression either by affecting mRNA stability when occurring in a gene's 3′-untranslated region or by changing transcription factor binding when occurring in the 5′-promoter region. A polymorphism does not have any effect on the protein product when it occurs within DNA regions that are not involved in gene transcription or translation but serves as the basis for genetic linkage analysis [1].

IntechOpen

The information on genetic polymorphisms facilitates to explain pathologic mechanisms and help in identifying individuals at risk. It also helps us to find novel targets for drug treatment. The protein tyrosine phosphatase non-receptor type 22 (*PTPN22*) gene is an important predisposing gene for human autoimmune diseases. The alterations in PTPN22 render a person susceptible and lead to the development of several autoimmune diseases. Many single nucleotide polymorphisms (SNPs) have been identified in PTPN22, but only one non-synonymous SNP has been intensively studied in relation to autoimmune diseases. This SNP C1858T (rs2476601) in exon 14 of the PTPN22 gene has been associated with a number of autoimmune diseases and considered as a risk factor due to significant production of autoantibodies [2, 3].

The PTPN22 C1858T variant has been studied in autoimmune diseases such as rheumatoid arthritis (RA), systemic lupus erythematosus (SLE), type 1 diabetes mellitus, juvenile idiopathic arthritis (JIA), inflammatory bowel disease (IBD) including Crohn's disease (CD) and ulcerative colitis (UC), antineutrophil cytoplasmic antibody (ANCA)-associated vasculitis, vitiligo, systemic sclerosis (SSc), Graves' disease (GD), myasthenia gravis (MG), Addison's disease, psoriasis, psoriatic arthritis (PsA), Behcet's disease (BD), endometriosis, autoimmune thyroid disease (AITD), giant cell arteritis (GCA), alopecia areata (AA), and Sjögren's syndrome. The association of PTPN22 C1858T genetic polymorphism is very significant and noteworthy in some autoimmune diseases, while in other it is less significant [3]. However, available literature on PTPN22 C1858T polymorphism and autoimmune diseases shows inconsistencies and ethnic variations exist.

2. *PTPN22* gene

PTPN22 gene is located on chromosomes 1p13.3–p13.1 and encodes a lymphoid-specific tyrosine phosphatase (Lyp). Lyp is an intracellular protein tyrosine phosphatase, bound to the SH3 domain of the C-terminal Src kinase (Csk) through a proline-rich motif. It is believed to suppress kinases mediating T-cell activation [4]. Lyp plays an important role in B-cell signaling, besides functioning as a negative regulator of T cells. It works in signaling cascade at various levels and targets several signaling intermediates involved in T-cell receptor signaling [5, 6]. After HLA, PTPN22 gene is the second-most important predisposing gene for human autoimmune diseases.

The minor allele 1858T in the *PTPN22* locus has a strong and consistent genetic association with autoimmune diseases. In PTPN22 C1858T (rs2476601), cytosine changes to thymidine at nucleotide 1858, resulting in an amino acid change from arginine to tryptophan at codon 620 (R620W), located in the polyproline-binding motif P1 [7, 8]. Yet there is no consensus whether C1858T polymorphism is a gain- or loss-of-function variant. The C1858T has been reported as a susceptibility locus associated with several autoimmune diseases. It was first reported in type 1 diabetes mellitus (T1DM) [7].

PTPN22 C1858T polymorphism has been suggested to increase Lyp protein activity which in turn inhibits T-cell signaling and results in a failure to delete autoreactive T cells during thymic selection. The association of this polymorphism is restricted to disorders that have a strong autoantibody component as it results in immune responses against autoantigens [8].

With the advent of new genotyping and molecular biology techniques, a huge amount of data are available for analysis. A large number of genes associated with diseases have been identified by the GWAS, candidate gene, and epidemiological studies. Therefore, the focus should be on the way genetic associations are reported. Even in the overlapping meta-analyses on the same topic, the limitations such as inclusion and exclusion criteria and number of included studies result in consistency of association results of genes, although the meta-analysis has been considered as a powerful approach to identify true-positive association of genes with disease.

The PTPN22 C1858T variant has been studied in several autoimmune or autoimmunity-related diseases in different ethnic populations worldwide.

3. Autoimmune diseases

Autoimmune diseases are pathological conditions identified by abnormal autoimmune responses and characterized by autoantibodies and T-cell responses to self-molecules by immune system reactivity. Human autoimmune diseases occur frequently (affecting in aggregate more than 5% of the population worldwide) and impose a significant burden of morbidity and mortality on the human population [9].

The etiology of autoimmune diseases involves both genetic and environmental factors. Familial clustering is known in autoimmune diseases with higher rate of concordance in monozygotic twins as compared to dizygotic twins [10–12]. Most autoimmune diseases are multigenic, with multiple susceptibility genes working in concert to produce the disease; however, a few autoimmune diseases are caused by mutations in a single gene. Even in such cases other genes modify the severity of disease. On the other hand, some individuals with these mutations do not manifest the disease.

The genetic polymorphisms also occur in normal population and are compatible with a normal immune function. However, when these polymorphisms occur with

Population	Case/controls	Genotype/allele/polymorphism	Association	References
Mexican	187/223	CT	Susceptible	[20]
Indian (Tamils)	264/264	CT	Susceptible	[25]
Indian (Gujarati)	126/140	C1858T	No association	[32]
English	165/304	C1858T	Susceptible	[29]
Romanian	–	T-allele	Susceptible	[30]
European* Asian	2094/3613	T-allele T-allele	Susceptible No association	[28]
Turkish	107/112	C1858T	No association	[27]
European* Asian	1800/3269	T-allele T-allele	Susceptible No association	[26]
Jordanian	55/85	C1858T	No association	[33]
Egyptian	100/120	C1858T	No association	[34]
Caucasian# European	1514/2813	C1858T	Susceptible	[31]

**Meta-analysis.*
#Genome-wide association study.

Table 1.
Association of PTPN22 C1858T polymorphism with vitiligo *susceptibility.*

other susceptibility genes, they develop autoimmunity [13, 14]. The extent of risk is not same for all such genes, and some of the genes confer a much higher level of risk than others [9].

The results of various association studies of PTPN22 C1858T variant with some of the autoimmune diseases are summarized in **Tables 1–18**.

Population	Case/controls	Genotype/allele/polymorphism	Association	References
Mexican	64/225	T-allele	Susceptible	[41]
Belgian-German	435/628	C1858T	Susceptible	[39]
English	196/507	C1858T	Susceptible	[38]
Mixed*	1129/1702	T and CT	Susceptible	[43]
Mixed*	365/173	C1858T	Susceptible	[42]
Egyptian	103/100	CT, TT	Susceptible	[40]
Iranian	69/69	T-allele	No association	[44]

**Meta-analysis.*

Table 2.
Association of PYPN22 C1858T polymorphism with alopecia *susceptibility.*

Population	Case/controls	Genotype/allele/polymorphism	Association	References
Saudi	106/200	T-allele, CT	Susceptible	[53]
German	375 + 418/376 + 561	C1858T	No association	[57]
English	647/566	C1858T	No association	[58]
Caucasian	1146	C1858T	No association	[59]
Mixed*	3334/5753	T-allele	No association	[56]
Mixed*	1448/1385	C1858T	No association	[55]
Cretan (Greek)	173/348	T-allele	No association	[60]

**Meta-analysis.*

Table 3.
Association of PTPN22 C1858T polymorphism with psoriasis *susceptibility.*

Population	Case/controls	Genotype/allele/polymorphism	Association	References
Toronto (admixed)	207/199	T-allele	Susceptible	[61]
Swedish	291/725	T-allele	Susceptible	[62]
Mixed#	1177/2155	C1858T	Susceptible	[63]
UK	455/595	C1858T	No association	[65]
Newfoundland	238/149	T-allele	No association	[61]
German	375/376	T-allele	No association	[66]

#Genome-wide association study.

Table 4.
Association of PTPN22 C1858T polymorphism with psoriatic arthritis *susceptibility.*

Population	Case/ controls	Genotype/allele/ polymorphism	Association	References
American (European ancestry)	647/751	C1858T	Susceptible	[67]
Australian	324/568	C1858T	Susceptible	[70]
Australian	413/690 1608/9284	C1858T	Susceptible in females	[71]
Greek	128/221	C1858T	Susceptible	[73]
Egyptian	60/40	T-allele	Susceptible	[75]
UK	661/595	C1858T	Susceptible	[65]
Czechs	130/400	T-allele	Susceptible	[72]
European	809/3535	C1858T	Susceptible	[69]
Norwegian	320/555	C1858T	Susceptible	[74]
Mixed*	4552/10,161	C1858T	Susceptible	[77]
Mixed*	4238/6012	C1858T	Susceptible	[76]
Finish	230	T-allele	No association	[78]
Hungarian	150/200	T-allele	No association	[79]

**Meta-analysis.*

Table 5.
Association of PTPN22 C1858T polymorphism with juvenile idiopathic arthritis *susceptibility.*

Population	Case/controls	Genotype/allele/polymorphism	Association	References
Spanish	826/1036	T-allele	Susceptible	[96]
Italian	396/477	T-allele	Susceptible	[92]
Turkish	323/426	C1858T	Susceptible	[97]
Colombian	298/308	T-allele	Susceptible	[86]
Colombian	413/434	T-allele	Susceptible	[87]
Egyptian	150/150	T-allele	Susceptible	[89]
Egyptian	394/398	C1858T	Susceptible	[90]
Egyptian	112/122	T-allele	Susceptible	[88]
Egyptian	100/114	C1858T	No association	[100]
Algerian	110/197	C1858T	Susceptible	[85]
Mexican	315/315	C1858T	Susceptible	[95]
Mexican	364/387	C1858T	Susceptible	[94]
Mexican	309/347	T-allele	Susceptible	[93]
UK	886/595	C1858T	Susceptible	[65]
Iranian	120/120	C1858T	Susceptible	[91]
Iranian	120/120	T-allele	Susceptible	[84]
Iranian	405/467	C1858T	No association	[101]
Chinese Han	358/564	C1858T	No association	[99]
Chinese-Yunnan	192/288	C1858T	No association	[98]

Population	Case/controls	Genotype/allele/polymorphism	Association	References
Caucasian* Asian*	27,205/27,677	C1858T C1858T	Susceptible No association	[103]
European* Asian and African	29 studies	C1858T C1858T	Susceptible No association	[104]
Mixed*	11,727/12,640	T-allele	Susceptible	[105]
Mixed*	3209/3692	C1858T	Susceptible	[106]
Mixed*	20,344/21,828	C1858T	Susceptible	[76]
Mixed*	13 studies	T-allele	Susceptible	[107]
Mixed*	17,961/18,611	C1858T	Susceptible	[102]
Mixed*	34 studies	C1858T	Susceptible	[108]
Mixed*	36 studies	T-allele	Susceptible	[2]

**Meta-analysis.*

Table 6.
Association of PTPN22 C1858T polymorphism with RA *susceptibility.*

Population	Case/ controls	Genotype/allele/ polymorphism	Association	References
Spanish	338/1036	T-allele	Susceptible	[96]
Swedish	571/1042	C1858T	Susceptible	[120]
American	525/1961	C1858T	Susceptible	[116]
Crete	328/427	C1858T	Susceptible	[119]
Colombian	94/434	T-allele	Susceptible	[87]
Colombian	143/308	T-allele	Susceptible	[86]
Polish	135/201	CT, T-allele	Susceptible	[122]
Polish	150/300	C1858T	Susceptible	[121]
Mixed*	6 studies	T-allele	susceptible	[107]
Mixed*	772/1092	C1858T	Susceptible	[126]
Mixed*	9120/11724	C1858T	Susceptible	[128]
Mixed*	11 studies	CT, TT	Susceptible	[125]
Mixed*	14 studies	T-allele	Susceptible	[2]
Mixed*	3868/7458	T-allele, TT	Susceptible	[127]
European-Americans	3936/3491	C1858T	Susceptible	[118]
Hispanics	1492/807	C1858T	No association	[118]
African-Americans	1527/1811	C1858T	No association	[118]
Asians	1265/1260	C1858T	No association	[118]
Egyptian	170/241	C1858T	Susceptible	[124]
Egyptian	40/20	CT	Susceptible	[123]
Egyptian	60/60	C1858T	No association	[133]
European-American	1680/1467	T-allele	Susceptible	[117]
Mexican	500/355	T-allele	Susceptible	[134]

Population	Case/ controls	Genotype/allele/ polymorphism	Association	References
Mexican mestizos	150/150	C1858T	No association	[130]
Turkish	158/155	C1858T	No association	[131]
Turkish	137/160	C1858T	No association	[132]
Chinese Han	713/672	C1858T	No association	[99]
Chinese	40/20	C1858T	No association	[129]

*Meta-analysis.

Table 7.
Association of PTPN22 C1858T polymorphism with SLE *susceptibility.*

Population	Case/controls	Genotype/allele/polymorphism	Association	References
Egyptian	60/60	C1858T	Susceptible	[133]
German	140/100	T-allele	Susceptible	[138]
Mixed*	3764/3328	C1858T	Susceptible	[139]
Japanese	456/221	T-allele	No association	[143]
Japanese	334/179	C1858T	No association	[144]
Korean	212/225	T-allele	No association	[145]
Polish	149/200	C1858T	No association	[147]
Jordanian Arab	204/2016	C1858T	No association	[146]

*Meta-analysis.

Table 8.
Association of PTPN22 C1858T polymorphism with AITD *susceptibility.*

Population	Case/controls	Genotype/allele/polymorphism	Association	References
Latin-American	83/336	C1858T	Susceptible	[148]
Polish	166/154	C1858T	Susceptible	[149]
Polish	290/310	T-allele	Susceptible	[150]
Polish	735/1216	C1858T	No association	[154]
English	768/768	C1858T	Susceptible	[140]
English	549/429	C1858T	Susceptible	[151]
English	901/833	C1858T	Susceptible	[152]
Mixed*	3 studies	T-allele	Susceptible	[2]
Mixed*	3764/3328	C1858T	Susceptible	[139]
Indian Kashmiri	135/150	C1858T	No association	[155]
Chinese Han#	5904/5866	C1858T	No association	[153]

*Meta-analysis.
#Genome-wide association study.

Table 9.
Association of PTPN22 C1858T polymorphism with Graves' disease *susceptibility.*

Population	Case/controls	Genotype/allele/ polymorphism	Association	Reference
Tunisian	164/100	C1858T	Susceptible	[163]
Moroccan	195/311	C1858T	No association	[167]
Spanish	1903CD, 1677UC/ 3111	C1858T	Protective to CD	[165]
New Zealanders	315/4081	C1858T	No association with CD	[168]
Czech	345/501	C1858T	No association	[169]
Canadian	455/190	C1858T	No association with CD	[170]
Canadian	249/207	T-allele	No association with CD	[171]
British	514/374	C1858T	No association	[172]
Spanish	1113/812	C1858T	No association	[173]
German	146	C1858T	No association with CD	[174]
Mixed*	8182/13356	C1858T	Susceptible to CD	[164]
Meta-analysis		C1858T	Protective to CD	[2]
Italian	649/256	C1858T	No association	[175]

**Meta-analysis.*

Table 10.
Association of PTPN22 C1858T polymorphism with IBD (CD + UC) *susceptibility.*

Population	Case/controls	Genotype/allele/ polymorphism	Association	References
Saudi	372/372	T-allele	Susceptible	[184]
German	220/239	C1858T	Susceptible	[185]
Egyptian	150/165	T-allele	Susceptible	[186]
Egyptian	120/120	T-allele	Susceptible	[187]
Kuwaiti Arabs	253/2014	T-allele	Susceptible	[188]
Chinese	202/240	C1858T	Susceptible	[189]
Chinese	364/719	C1858T	No association	[178]
Brazilian	612/792	C1858T	Susceptible	[190]
Brazilian	205/308	C1858T	Susceptible	[191]
Polish	215/236	C1858T	Susceptible	[192]
Polish	147/327	C1858T	Susceptible	[193]
Russian	27/62 families	C1858T	Susceptible	[194]
Croatian	102/193	T-allele	Susceptible	[195]
Caucasian	140/100	T-allele	Susceptible	[138]
Caucasian	8677	C1858T	Susceptible	[196]
Caucasian	113	C1858T	Susceptible	[197]
Czechs	372/400	T-allele	Susceptible	[72]
Iranian (Azeri)	160/271	T-allele	Susceptible	[72]

Population	Case/controls	Genotype/allele/ polymorphism	Association	References
Iranian	99/100	C1858T	Susceptible	[84]
Iranian	144/197	C1858T	No association	[181]
Estonian	170/230	T-allele	Susceptible	[198]
Italian	271/89	C1858T	Susceptible	[199]
Spanish	316/554	T-allele	Susceptible	[200]
Colorado	753/662	CT, TT	Susceptible	[201]
Colombian	110/308	T-allele	Susceptible	[86]
Colombian	197 families	C1858T	Susceptible	[202]
International children	257	C1858T	Associated with proinsulin levels	[203]
Mixed*	6 studies	C1858T	Susceptible	[107]
Mixed*	19,495/25,341	C1858T	Susceptible	[204]
Mixed*	22,485/35,292	C1858T	Susceptible in Caucasian	[205]
Mixed*	11 studies	T-allele	Susceptible in European	[206]
Mixed*	16,240/17,997	C1858T	Susceptible	[207]
Mixed*	8869/20,829	C1858T	Susceptible	[208]
Mixed*	10 studies	C1858T	Susceptible	[209]
Indian	145/210	T-allele	Susceptible	[210]
Indian	129/109	C1858T	No association	[180]
Greek	130/135	C1858T	No association	[179]

*Meta-analysis.

Table 11.
Association of PTPN22 C1858T polymorphism with T1DM *susceptibility.*

Population	Case/ controls	Genotype/allele/ polymorphism	Association	References
French	659/504	T-allele	Susceptible	[216]
French	121/103	C1858T	No association	[218]
Mixed White, Black, Hispanic	1120/716	C1858T	Susceptible	[217]
Caucasian	3422/3638	C1858T	Susceptible	[214]
Mixed*	4367/4771	C1858T	Susceptible	[107]
Columbian	101/434	T-allele	No association	[87]
Spanish	54/55	C1858T	No association	[219]

*Meta-analysis.

Table 12.
Association of PTPN22 C1858T polymorphism with systemic sclerosis *susceptibility.*

Population	Case/controls	Genotype/allele/polymorphism	Association	References
Swedish	409/1557	C1858T	Susceptible	[228]
German	125/301	C1858T	Susceptible	[229]
European	649/	C1858T	Susceptible	[230]
Mixed*	2802/3730	C1858T	Susceptible	[221]
Hungarian, German	282/379	T-allele	Susceptible	[231]
French	470/296	C1858T	Susceptible	[232]
European#	532/2128	C1858T	Susceptible	[235]
Chinese	79/50	C1858T	No association	[2]
Turkish	416/293	C1858T	No association	[234]
Italian	356/439	C1858T	No association	[233]

*Meta-analysis.
#Genome-wide association study.

Table 13.
Association of PTPN22 C1858T polymorphism with myasthenia gravis *susceptibility.*

Population	Case/controls	Genotype/allele/polymorphism	Association	References
Spanish	404/1517	C1858T	No association	[243]
Turkish	134/177	C1858T	No association	[242]
UK and Middle East	270/203	C1858T	Protective	[241]
Mixed*	1922/11,505	C1858T	No association	[76]

*Meta-analysis.

Table 14.
Association of PTPN22 (C1858T) polymorphism with Behcet's disease *susceptibility.*

Population	Case/controls	Genotype/allele/polymorphism	Association	Reference
Italian	132/232	C1858T	Susceptible	[252]
Italian	132/359	T-allele	Susceptible	[253]
Italian	130/250	C1858T	Susceptible	[254]
Brazilian	140/180	C1858T	Susceptible	[255]
Mixed*	971/1181	T-allele	Susceptible	[246]
Polish	171/310	C1858T	No association	[248]

*Meta-analysis.

Table 15.
Association of PTPN22 C1858T polymorphism with endometriosis *susceptibility.*

Population	Case/controls	Genotype/allele/polymorphism	Association	References
German	199/399	T-allele	Susceptible	[259]
British	641/9115	C1858T	Susceptible	[260]
Italian	344/945	C1858T	Susceptible	[261]

Population	Case/controls	Genotype/allele/polymorphism	Association	References
Mixed*	1399/9934	C1858T	Susceptible in White	[262]
Mixed*	1922/11,505	C1858T	Susceptible	[76]

*Meta-analysis.

Table 16.
Association of PTPN22 C1858T polymorphism with antineutrophil cytoplasmic antibody (ANCA)-associated vasculitis *susceptibility.*

Population	Case/ Controls	Genotype/allele/ polymorphism	Association	References
Spanish	95/229	C1858T	No association	[263]
Spanish, German, Norwegian	911/8136	C1858T	Susceptible	[265]
European	1651/ 15,306	C1858T	Susceptible	[266]
Australian	209/455	T-allele	Susceptible	[267]

Table 17.
Association of PTPN22 C1858T polymorphism with giant cell arteritis *susceptibility.*

Population	Case/controls	Genotype/allele/polymorphism	Association	References
Norwegian	332/990	T-allele	Susceptible	[269]
UK and Polish	338/665	T-allele	Susceptible	[270]
English	104/429	C1858T	Susceptible	[151]
Mixed*	6 studies	T-allele	Susceptible	[2]
German	121/239	C1858T	No association	[185]
Mixed*	2 studies	C1858T	No association	[107]

*Meta-analysis.

Table 18.
Association of PTPN22 C1858T polymorphism with Addison's disease *susceptibility.*

4. Vitiligo

Vitiligo is an acquired, autoimmune skin disorder characterized by melanocyte loss resulting into progressive depigmentation of the skin and hair [15, 16]. The prevalence of vitiligo varies considerably with ethnicity and it affects 0.1–2% of the population worldwide [15, 17]. Vitiligo is associated with an elevated risk of several other autoimmune diseases [18–20].

Vitiligo commonly shows familial aggregation and multifactorial mode of inheritance. It is a polygenic disease, and several genes related to autoimmunity have been reported to be associated with the pathogenesis of vitiligo [20–25].

Various published reports on PTPN22 C1858T polymorphism support the association of the T-allele and vitiligo susceptibility in different ethnic populations (**Table 1**). However, available literature on the PTPN22 C1858T polymorphism and vitiligo susceptibility is inconsistent [25–28]. It has been reported to be a risk factor for vitiligo in English, Romanian, North American, Mexican, and South Indian Tamil populations [20, 25, 29, 30]. PTPN22 C1858T polymorphism is strongly associated with vitiligo susceptibility in Saudis also [in press]. A genome-wide association study indicates that PTPN22 C1858T is associated with vitiligo in European-derived white patients [Jin et al. 2010]. A meta-analysis utilizing data from different ethnicities shows an association of PTPN22 C1858T with vitiligo in European but not in Asian population [28].

In contrast, no significant association of PTPN22 C1858T polymorphism with susceptibility to generalized vitiligo was found in Indian Gujarat population, Jordanian, Egyptian female, and Turkish population [27, 32–34]. Available literature shows that the variant of PTPN22 C1858T is responsible for increased risk of vitiligo in Caucasian patients; however, among non-Caucasians/Asians, inconsistency exits, and even the two populations of same country differ in association of PTPN22 C1858T with vitiligo indicating the role of ethnicity. The heterozygous CT genotype of the PTPN22 C1858T has a strong association with non-segmental vitiligo in South Indian Tamils, while there is no association of this polymorphism in Indian Gujarat population [25, 32]. This difference in the results of this polymorphism in Asians or non-Caucasians can be attributed to ethnic differences.

5. Alopecia areata (AA)

AA is a dermatological condition in which hair is lost from certain or all areas of the body, typically from certain areas of the scalp, more frequent in young ones [35]. The characteristic feature of AA is circular or oval bald spots which may progress and spread to the entire scalp (alopecia totalis) or entire body (alopecia universalis). Sometimes hair loss is localized to the sides and lower back of the scalp which is known as alopecia ophiasis [36]. The prevalence of AA in the general population varies between 0.1 and 6.9% depending on the ethnic group [37].

Alopecia areata is an autoimmune disease mediated by T cells to the hair follicles. There are enough evidences indicating that AA is a complex multigenetic trait with components of inherited predisposition. Molecular biology studies have led to the identification of a number of candidate genes in humans that confer susceptibility to AA. Recently, PTPN22 gene has been reported to be an additional immunoregulatory gene associated with AA. PTPN22 C1858T polymorphism has been associated with susceptibility of AA in Belgian, English, Egyptian, German, and Mexican populations (**Table 2**) [38–43]. Two meta-analyses have also indicated an association with AA susceptibility [42, 43]. However, no association of PTPN22 C1858T has been found in Iranian patients [44].

6. Psoriasis

Psoriasis is a chronic, complex autoimmune disease with characteristic reddish patches covered by silvery-white scales. It affects approximately 120–180 million people worldwide [45]. The prevalence of psoriasis varies significantly depending mainly on race, geographical location, genetics, environmental factors, and ethnicity [46–50].

The etiology of psoriasis involves both genetic and environmental factors indicating a multifactorial nature. Moreover, a number of characteristic features of psoriasis are also found in other autoimmune diseases indicating a common etiology [51, 52].

Though the pathogenesis of psoriasis and comorbidities has been studied at the molecular level and a number of gene loci have been associated with susceptibility/severity of psoriasis [50–53], genes identified till date to be associated with it do not fully account for it. Psoriasis is highly heritable, and it has been suggested in several association studies that skin barrier function, innate and adaptive immunity, and gene-gene and gene-environment interactions are involved in the pathogenesis of psoriasis [52].

Recently an association of T-allele of the PTPN22 C1858T with susceptibility to psoriasis in Saudi population was reported (**Table 3**) [53]. Earlier it has been suggested that *PTPN22* may be among the true psoriasis susceptibility risk genes [54]. However, another study analyzed 15 SNPs from 7 putative psoriasis-risk genes and could not find any significant association of PTPN22 C1858T polymorphism with psoriasis. On the other hand, they found a significant association with another polymorphism (rs3789604) in *PTPN22* gene and suggested that *PTPN22* is one of the significant risk genes for psoriasis [55]. Chen and Chang [56] reported a strong association of PTPN22 + 1858T allele with PsA but no association with psoriasis and suggested that attention should be given to the studies dealing with gene-environment interaction besides keeping in consideration the clinical heterogeneity of the disease and population stratification.

Earlier Hüffmeier et al. [57] found gender variations in susceptibility of PTPN22 (+1858T allele) with psoriasis and suggested that other susceptibility locus/loci within noncoding regions of *PTPN22* or its proximity might exist and act independently as a risk factor. They excluded the direct link of T-allele in psoriasis susceptibility in German psoriasis patients.

7. Psoriatic arthritis

PsA is a chronic inflammatory arthritis associated with psoriasis. PsA is a chronic skin and joint condition that considerably affects patient's quality of life. PsA is a complex disease with environmental and genetic risk factors contributing to it. Several studies have demonstrated different associations of genetic polymorphisms in the pathogenic process of PsA.

PTPN22 C1858T polymorphism has also been strongly associated with PsA (**Table 4**) in Toronto admix and Swedish population [61, 62]. Several non-HLA loci including *PTPN22* have been suggested to affect the susceptibility to PsA [63, 64]. A complete genetic overlap has been suggested between psoriasis and PsA susceptibility loci as about a third of people who have psoriasis gets PsA. It has been noticed that subjects with severe psoriasis have a greater chance of getting PsA and about 40% of patients with PsA have relatives with it or with psoriasis, while other earlier studies reported no association of PTPN22 C1858T polymorphism and PsA in Newfoundland, the UK, and German Caucasian [57, 61, 65]. Though no significant differences were observed in allele distribution with different manifestations of disease, there is gender difference, and male PsA patients has higher frequency of T-allele than in the subgroup of female patients [66].

8. Juvenile idiopathic arthritis

JIA is the most common inflammatory disease of the joints in children. Its etiology is complex and involves both genetic and environmental factors. It has been suggested that genetic factors play a significant role in the susceptibility to JIA [67]. While associations between JIA and variants in HLA are well established, non-HLA genetic variants also play a role in JIA susceptibility and have increasingly been identified by genome-wide and candidate gene studies [68, 69]. Many of the genetic associations have been confirmed recently by the International JIA Immunochip consortium, and several novel loci have also been identified showing a genome-wide association.

Several reports indicate that PTPN22 C1858T polymorphism has been consistently associated with JIA (**Table 5**). PTPN22 C1858T polymorphism is associated with JIA in Australians [70, 71], Americans of European ancestry [67], Czech [72], Europeans [69], Greek [73], Norwegians [74], UK population [65], and Egyptians [75]. Two separate meta-analyses also indicated that PTPN22 C1858T is associated with susceptibility to JIA [76, 77]. However, it is not associated with JIA in Finish and Hungarian patients [78, 79]. These variations may be due to ethnic variations; however, methodological error in genotyping cannot be ruled out.

9. Rheumatoid arthritis

RA is a chronic autoimmune disorder of bone joints caused by the complex interplay between several factors like body physiology and the environment with genetic background [80, 81]. RA is characterized by synovial inflammation, hyperplasia, cartilage and bone destruction, autoantibody production (rheumatoid factor), anticyclic citrullinated peptide (CCP), and the decreased quality of life [82]. Its prevalence is approximately 0.51% worldwide and afflicts people of all races.

RA shares a number of pathogenic mechanisms with other autoimmune disorders. More than 100 loci have been associated with RA as shown in a meta-analysis of GWAS. Out of these majority (97%) are located in the noncoding region, and the remaining 3% are in various non-HLA genes including PTPN22 (Trp620Arg) [83].

Several studies have been performed on the association of PTPN22 C1858T variants with RA susceptibility in different ethnic populations (**Table 6**). Various studies have demonstrated that allelic heterogeneity distribution has an increasing north-south gradient in the frequencies of the 1858T alleles in different European populations [84]. PTPN22 C1858T polymorphism has been associated with susceptibility to RA in Algerian [85], Colombian [86, 87], Egyptian [88–90], Iranian [84, 91], Italian [92], Mexican [93–95], Spanish [96], Turkish [97], and UK Caucasian populations [65].

On the other hand, some studies reported that it is not associated with RA in Chinese [98, 99], Egyptian [100], and Iranian populations [101]. A number of meta-analyses have also shown that T-allele of PTPN22 C1858T is associated with RA susceptibility in Caucasians but not in Asians and Africans (**Table 6**) [102–104]. The different allele frequency of T-allele is very important in determining the population attributable risk of this allele for the autoimmune diseases in different populations. It also affects any suggested screening or predictive testing protocol for these diseases [101]. The absence of this association in Asians undermines the importance of this locus as a susceptibility locus for the RA and other autoimmune diseases.

10. Systemic lupus erythematosus

SLE is a heterogeneous autoimmune inflammatory disease characterized by loss of self-tolerance with hyperactivation of autoreactive T and B cells with a predominance of Th2 inflammatory response [109]. The SLE incidence rate varies from 1 to 10 per 100,000 person/years, and the prevalence varies from 20 to 70 per 100,000 persons. SLE affects more than 300,000 people in the United States (USA) and millions worldwide [110]. It is characterized by multisystem involvement, autoantibody formation, and dysregulation of the complement system. The onset of SLE is postulated to be triggered by environmental and hormonal factors in genetically susceptible individuals [111, 112].

The genetic contribution to the development of SLE is considerably high, which is estimated to be 66% of heritability in twin studies. Genome-wide association studies (GWASs) have greatly improved our understanding of the genetic basis of SLE [113]. A high-density SNP analysis has identified and facilitated to focus on disease-associated loci where patients and healthy controls exhibit different frequencies of trait-associated alleles which are potential disease-causal variants or their proxies [113]. To date, about 100 SLE susceptibility loci have been identified, mostly in European and Asian populations [112], explaining the heritability of SLE up to around 30% [114, 115]. The highly polygenic etiology of SLE is supported by a large number of disease-associated loci that have modest effect sizes but surpass the genome-wide significance threshold for the genetic association with SLE as reviewed by Kwon et al. [112].

PTPN22 C1858T polymorphism has been associated with the pathogenesis of SLE in various populations (**Table 7**). This polymorphism is significantly associated with susceptibility to SLE in American [116–118], Columbian [86, 87], Crete [119], Spanish [96], Swedish [120], Polish [121, 122], Egyptian populations [123, 124].

Several meta-analyses also indicated that PTPN22 C1858T polymorphism is associated with SLE susceptibility [2, 107, 125–128]. On the other hand, it is not associated with SLE in Asians [118], Chinese [99, 129], Hispanics, African-Americans [118], Mexican mestizos [130], and Turkish patients [131, 132].

11. Autoimmune thyroid disease

Autoimmune thyroid disease (AITD) is a complex disease which includes GD and Hashimoto's thyroiditis (HT). Its susceptibility is influenced by both genetic and environmental factors. The interaction of specific susceptibility genes and environmental exposures have been associated with AITD [135]. Both GD and HT are characterized by the production of thyroid autoantibodies and the invasion of thyroid lymphocytes. AITD is found in 5% of the general population and is one of the most prevalent autoimmune diseases. The incidence of GD and HT is influenced by genetic factors as well as environmental factors including geographical locations [136]. Approximately 37% of families with AITD exhibit either of these two disorders [137].

Previous molecular studies on genetic etiology of AITD have expanded the field of thyroid autoimmunity. Previous studies have shown that PTPT22 C1858T is associated with AITD [138, 139] (**Table 8**). Some reports have indicated a positive correlation [140–142], while others have indicated no correlation between PTPN22 C1858T and AITD in Japanese [143, 144], Korean [145], Jordanian, [146], and Polish populations [147].

PTPN22 C1858T polymorphism has been associated with GD (**Table 9**). It is susceptible to GD in Latin-American [148], Polish [149, 150], and English Caucasian populations [140, 151, 152]. Two separate meta-analyses confirmed the association of PTPN22 + 1858C/T polymorphism with Graves' disease [2, 139]. However, some reports have indicated no correlation between PTPN22 + 1858C/T and Graves' disease in Chinese Han, Polish, and Indian Kashmiri populations [153–155].

Jacobson et al. [156] reported that the PTPN22 + 1858C/T is related to the occurrence of HT. Another variant in PTPN22 gene has been found to be associated with HT using whole-exome sequencing [157] indicating the role of *PTPN22* in autoimmune thyroid disease. However, the functional mechanism involved in the association remains to be found out.

12. Inflammatory bowel disease

IBD is a complex, multifactorial, chronic inflammatory disorder of the gastrointestinal tract in which immune dysregulation caused by genetic and/or environmental factors plays an important role. IBD refers to two chronic inflammatory disorders of the gastrointestinal tract: UC and CD.

The IBD is a complex autoimmune disease. Its etiology is characterized by immune dysregulation caused by genetic and/or environmental factors [158, 159]. A genetically susceptible person develops IBD as a result of the immunogenic responses against environmental factors and/or microbes inhabiting the distal ileum and colon. It is believed that genetic factors contribute significantly to the pathogenesis of IBD [160–162]. Genome-wide scans performed in patients with IBD have failed to find a major unique susceptibility locus and have prompted the general agreement that these diseases are polygenic entities in which several genes may contribute to susceptibility [162].

Sfar et al. [163] reported an association of PTPN22 C1858T polymorphism with IBD in Tunisian patients. Recently a meta-analysis utilizing 8182 patients and 13,356 controls indicated that this is associated with CD susceptibility only and there is no association with UC [164]. No association of PTPN22 C1858T polymorphism with IBD was found in British, Canadian, Czech, German, Italian, Moroccan, New Zealander, and Spanish populations (**Table 10**). Another study on Spanish patients showed that this polymorphism is protective to CD while there is no association with UC [165]. A meta-analysis also indicated that PTPN22 C1858T polymorphism is associated with reduced susceptibility to CD with no association with UC [2]. Despite the association of PTPN22 C1858T SNP with CD and several different autoimmune disorders, a role for this polymorphism in susceptibility to IBD does not establish.

Thus, it is plausible that this genetic discrepancy in PTPN22 influences a range of diseases in which the phenotypic spectrum includes an aberrant or hyperactive immune response [5, 166]. However, these variations in the association reports of PTPN22 C1858T polymorphism with IBD may be due to ethnic variations in genetic makeup of the different populations. It has been suggested that the presence of T-allele of PTPN22 C1858T makes an individual susceptible to autoimmune diseases by helping the production of antibodies associated with these diseases, resulting in the disease development [116].

13. Type 1 diabetes mellitus

Type 1 diabetes is an autoimmune disease in which the insulin-producing cells are attacked by the body's defense system resulting in no insulin or very little insulin production. Although the exact cause of the T1DM is not clear yet, it has been associated with both genetic and environmental factors. It usually develops in children or young adults but can affect people of all age group. The patient will die if there is no access to insulin. Therefore, daily injection of insulin is required to control the blood glucose levels in patients with T1DM.

The International Diabetes Federation (IDF) has reported that there were 382 million people living with diabetes worldwide in 2013 and this number is expected to rise to 592 million by 2035 [176]. Most people with diabetes live in low- and middle-income countries, where rapid changes in lifestyle have increased the prevalence of diabetes, cardiovascular diseases, and cancer, and these countries are expected to experience the greatest increase in cases of diabetes in the next 20 years. The global prevalence of diabetes was reported as 8.8% of the world's population (95% confidence interval 7.2–11.3%) in 2017, and it is expected to increase to 9.9% in 2045 [177]. At present in every seventh second, someone dies from diabetes or its complications. Fifty percent of these deaths are under the age of 60 years.

According to a report, 424.9 million people were having diabetes worldwide in 2017 which is expected to increase to 628.6 million people in 2045. The prevalence of diabetes is continuously increasing since the IDF Diabetes Atlas first was launched in 2000, and about 50% of the diabetes cases remain undiagnosed especially in developing countries which is a matter of concern [177].

A positive association between PTPN22 C1858 T polymorphism and susceptibility to the development of T1DM has been reported in a large number of studies from several populations (**Table 11**) with the exception of a few such as a single study from Chinese [178], Greek [179], Indian [180], and Iranian populations [181] where no association was found.

The review by Prezioso et al. [182] evaluated the role of the PTPN22 C1858 T in the prognosis of disease. On the basis of the potential role of C1858 T as a target for tertiary prevention trials and new therapeutic strategies, such as the Lyp inhibitors, they suggested that PTPN22 can be a promising target for therapeutic interventions and identification of at-risk subjects in autoimmune diseases such as T1DM.

It has been shown that several SNPs could potentially contribute to susceptibility to various autoimmune disorders including T1DM. However, 1858C/T SNP is the most stable, where T-allele correlates with T1DM (**Table 11**) [7, 142, 152, 183]. Habib et al. [211] demonstrate a role of PTPN22 1858T in signaling defects in both transitional and naïve B cells in healthy subjects resulting in an increased resistance to BCR-driven apoptosis in these cells and peripheral reservoir of autoreactive cells [212].

14. Systemic sclerosis

SSc is a complex disease with an autoimmune origin in which extensive fibrosis, vascular alterations, and autoantibodies against various cellular antigens are among the principal features [213]. Although the etiopathogenesis is not yet well understood, the results of numerous genetic association studies support genetic contributions as an important factor to SSc.

SSc occurs in persons who are genetically predisposed and have faced specific environmental factors with or without other randomly distributed factors [214, 215]. It has been consistently associated with the major histocompatibility complex variants. Non-HLA genes associated with immunity have also been associated with SSc susceptibility [214].

In spite of these findings, the complete genetic background of SSc, the nature of its genetic determinants, and how they contribute to SSc susceptibility and clinical manifestations are poorly understood. Interestingly, PTPN22 has emerged as an important genetic risk factor for human autoimmunity. The PTPN22 C1858T polymorphism in SSc has also been investigated and shows a trend of association (**Table 12**). It has been associated with SSc susceptibility in French [216], Caucasian [214], and White, Black, and Hispanic American [217]. A meta-analysis showed that PTPN22 1858T is susceptible to SSc [107]. Some other report shows the absence of any association between this polymorphism and SSc in French [218], Columbian [87], and Spanish [219].

15. Myasthenia gravis

MG is an antibody-mediated autoimmune disease against antigens at the neuromuscular junction. Both genetic and environmental factors contribute to the susceptibility of MG. The annual incidence of MG is reported to be 0.25–4 patients per 100,000 population, with the first peak of onset around the second and third decades of life and the second peak around the fifth and sixth decades [220, 221]. The exact mechanism of the autoimmunity in MG is unknown. It is caused mostly by the autoantibodies directed toward the skeletal muscle acetylcholine receptor (AChR), but there are cases in which autoimmune attack targets non-AChR components of the postsynaptic muscle endplate [222–225]. It has been suggested that genetic factors might play an important role in the development of MG [226–227]. Some studies showed that PTPN22 C1858T polymorphism is associated with MG risk (**Table 13**).

PTPN22 C1858T polymorphism is associated with MG susceptibility in Swedish [228], German [229], European [230], Hungarian [231], and French patients [232]. However, the association between this polymorphism and the risk of MG was controversial and inconclusive in Chinese, Italian, and Turkish patients [2, 233, 234].

16. Behcet's diseases

BD is characterized by recurrent orogenital ulcers, cutaneous inflammation, and uveitis. It is a chronic autoimmune/inflammatory disorder with typical mucocutaneous and ocular manifestations. It also targets musculoskeletal, nervous, vascular, and gastrointestinal systems [236]. The prevalence of BD varies with geographical locations. It is more prevalent in countries along the silk route, particularly in the East Asia and the Middle East. Prevalence is highest in Turkey, followed by Egypt, Morocco, Iraq, Saudi Arabia, Japan, Iran, Korea, and China [237, 238]. Available reports indicate that autoimmunity, genetic factors, and environmental factors are involved in the pathogenesis of BD; however, the specific etiology remains to be determined [236, 239, 240].

Being an autoimmune disease, BD is considered to be affected by PTPN22 C1858T polymorphism. However, there is no significant association of this gene in susceptibility to BD (**Table 14**). Baranathan et al. [241] suggested that PTPN22 C1858T is inversely associated with BD in the UK population indicating its protective role in BD. However, this does not hold for Middle Eastern patients in whom PTPN22 C1858T expression does not associate with BD, possibly due to a very low prevalence of the polymorphism in this population.

The prevalence of PTPN22 C1858T is very low in the general population, and the absence of any correlation with BD indicates that PTPN22 C1858T polymorphism has a limited role in the pathogenesis of autoimmunity [242]. Recently Ortiz-Fe rnández [243] also could not find any association of PTPN22 C1858T polymorphism with BD in Spanish patients.

17. Endometriosis

Endometriosis is a chronic inflammatory disease and one of the most common benign gynecological disorders. It is a condition in which a tissue that is histologically similar to the endometrium, with glands and/or stroma, grows outside the uterine cavity [244]. It presents a multisystem involvement affecting several organs, most commonly in the peritoneum and pelvis, especially the ovaries, and less often in the rectovaginal septum. This results in pelvic pain, dysmenorrhea, and infertility [245].

Although various hypotheses have been proposed to explain the etiology of endometriosis, the explanation of symptoms and presence of ectopic endometrial tissue and stroma at various sites is not very clear [246].

The etiology of endometriosis is complex and characterized by genetic and environmental factors similar to other autoimmune diseases. The immunological changes such as an increase in the number and cytotoxicity of macrophages, increase in the activity of B lymphocytes, abnormalities in the functions and concentrations of B and T lymphocytes, and reduction in the number or the activity of natural killer cells have been indicated in endometriosis. Anti-endometrial and anti-ovary antibodies have been also found in endometriosis [247]. As genetic factors and immunological predispositions are involved in the etiology of the disease, therefore the variants of genes associated with autoimmune diseases are possible candidates for endometriosis development [247]. PTPN22 C1858T polymorphism and its association with endometriosis have been studied in only three populations (Brazilian, Italian, and Polish) so far (**Table 15**).

The PTPN22 C1858T polymorphism has been reported to be associated with altered risk of endometriosis in Italian and Brazilian populations, but no significant association was found in Polish patients. However, on exploratory analyses Płoski et al. [248] suggested that the T-allele and the TT genotype may be associated with the prevalence of double positivity for antinuclear antibody (ANA) and anti-cardiolipin autoantibody (ACA).

A meta-analysis showed overall increased risk associations of up to 5.6-fold in endometriosis. In the presence of endometriosis, the PTPN22 C1858T polymorphism may cooperate with clinical and genetic factors to influence the course of disease and immune reactions. These cooperative interactions could result in a statistical association between PTPN22 C1858T and endometriosis [246].

The lymphoid tyrosine phosphatase enzyme is encoded by *PTPN22* gene and is a regulator of signaling through the T-cell receptor and forms a complex with the kinase Csk in T cells. The variant of PTPN22 C1858T polymorphism does not bind kinases properly and results in a gain-of-function enzyme [246, 249, 250]. The increased inhibition of T-cell receptor signaling caused by the PTPN22 C1858T polymorphism could predispose toward autoimmunity, either by affecting the thymic deletion of autoreactive T cells or by affecting the development or function of peripheral regulatory T cells [251].

18. Antineutrophil cytoplasmic antibody-associated vasculitis

Antineutrophil cytoplasmic antibody (ANCA)-associated vasculitis (AAV) is an uncommon inflammatory disease, characterized by inflammation in small- to medium-sized vessels, necrosis, and association with detectable circulating ANCAs. Though the manifestations in the lungs and kidneys are common, any organ or system can be affected. AAV refers to a group of small-vessel vasculitis, including granulomatosis with polyangiitis (GPA, formerly known as Wegener's granulomatosis), microscopic polyangiitis (MPA), and eosinophilic GPA (EGPA, formerly Churg-Strauss syndrome) [256].

AAV is a complex disease with both genetic and environmental factors involved in pathogenesis [257]. There is increasing evidence that susceptibility loci are shared between autoimmune diseases. The candidate gene association studies and the GWASs have shown the genetic basis of AAV. The significant association of AAV with HLA polymorphisms has confirmed the central role of autoimmunity in the development of AAV. All the three main subtypes mentioned above have been reported to be associated with distinct HLA variants [258].

The role of PTPN22 C1858T in AAV provided the basis for the three main PTPN22 genetic association studies performed so far (**Table 16**). The first, which included a German cohort, showed an association of this variant with the disease; the association was even more significant in the ANCA-positive subgroup [259]. This result has been subsequently replicated in two independent cohorts of British [260] and Italian AAV patients [261]. However, the study on Italian patients showed that the association is restricted to the GPA patients only, as almost similar frequency of the T-allele of PTPN22 C1858T was found in the MPA or the EGPA patients and controls.

Three independent meta-analyses indicated that PTPN22 C1858T polymorphism is significantly associated with susceptibility of AAV in Caucasian population [76, 262].

19. Giant cell arteritis

GCA is a form of vasculitis. It is very common in elderly people and may cause blindness and stroke [263]. The environmental, infectious, and genetic risk factors have been associated with GCA development; however, the pathogenesis is not clear yet. PTPN22 is a gene of interest which is proposed to be an "archetypal non-HLA autoimmunity gene" [251, 264]. The T-allele of a functional PTPN22 C1858T polymorphism has been reported to be associated with biopsy-proven GCA in Spanish patients (**Table 17**), with supporting data from three replicate Northern European studies [265]. Recently, this observation has been extended with additional patients and controls and studies encompassing European, Scandinavian, UK, and American patients [266], though an earlier report from Spanish patients does not support the potential involvement of PTPN22 gene polymorphism in the susceptibility or clinical expression of GCA [263].

Though Lester et al. [267] could not find any significant difference in the distribution of alleles and genotypes of PTPN22 C1858T polymorphism between patients and control groups, they suggested that there is a significant association between the minor allele of PTPN22 C1858T polymorphism and GCA.

20. Autoimmune Addison's disease (AAD)

AAD occurs due to autoimmune destruction of the adrenal cortex. Approximately half of the patients have additional autoimmune components. The prevalence of AAD varies from 110 to 144 cases per million in the developed countries. In adult patients, AAD is the most common etiological form (80%), followed by post-tuberculosis AD (10–15%) and vascular, neoplastic, or rare genetic forms (5%) [268]. AAD commonly coexists with thyroid autoimmunity and/or type I diabetes and is called as autoimmune polyendocrine syndrome type II (APS II).

Several genetic determinants have long been suspected to be involved in various autoimmune diseases. PTPN22 C1858T polymorphism has been studied in AAD patients with inconsistent results (**Table 18**). Velaga et al. [151] reported an association for the T-allele in patients from northeast England, whereas Kahles et al. [185] found no association in German patients. This inconsistency may be due to small sample size. The 1858T allele is associated with susceptibility to AAD in Norwegians [269], UK cohort, and the Polish population [270]. Meta-analysis of the results, together with those from three other populations, showed that the 1858T allele is associated with AAD susceptibility.

Confounding factors must be considered particularly when polymorphisms identified in one study cannot be duplicated in a similar ethnic group. One confounding factor is population stratification. This may occur with an unbalanced ethnic admixture.

It is clear that the inheritance of a coding variant of *PTPN22* gene is associated with increased susceptibility to autoimmunity. The mechanism by which the PTPN22 C1858T variant modulates disease risk has been studied. PTPN22 is capable of both enzymatic activities and adaptor functions. It exerts its effects in multiple biochemical pathways and cell types. PTPN22 regulates signaling through both antigen and innate immune receptors. It is involved in the development and activation of lymphocyte, establishment of tolerance, and innate immune cell-mediated host defense and immunoregulation. The PTPN22 C1858T variant protein is involved in the pathogenesis of autoimmunity at multiple levels. The action of PTPN22 C1858T during immature B-cell selection disrupts the establishment of a tolerant B-cell repertoire and alters mature T-cell responsiveness. When an autoimmune attack initiates tissue injury, the TPN22C1858T fosters inflammation by regulating the level of cytokines produced by a myeloid cell.

21. Conclusion

The PTPN22 C1858T is one of the strongest and most consistent genetic associations with autoimmune diseases. However, available literature on PTPN22 C1858T polymorphism and autoimmune diseases shows ethnic variations. It is conceivable that the relation of any locus with the autoimmune disease will be small as interactions between gene and gene and gene and environment might also be operating. Further well-designed studies from different populations and cohorts to detect small genetic risk will help in drawing better conclusion on the development of autoimmune diseases. Therefore, further genetic studies on patients suffering from various autoimmune diseases from different ethnicities and PTPN22 gene polymorphisms are expected to help better understand the pathogenesis and will contribute to the development of more targeted therapies and biomarkers.

Acknowledgements

Authors wish to thank the MSD administration for facilities and support.

Conflict of interest

No conflicts of interests.

Author details

Ghaleb Bin Huraib[1], Fahad Al Harthi[2], Misbahul Arfin[3]
and Abdulrahman Al-Asmari[3]*

1 Medical Services Department for Armed Forces, Riyadh, Saudi Arabia

2 Department of Dermatology, Prince Sultan Military Medical City, Riyadh, Saudi Arabia

3 Scientific Research Center, Medical Services Department for Armed Forces, Riyadh, Saudi Arabia

*Address all correspondence to: abdulrahman.alasmari@gmail.com
and misbahularfin@yahoo.com

References

[1] Weber JL, Broman KW. Genotyping for human whole-genome scans: Past, present, and future. Advances in Genetics. 2001;**42**:77-96. DOI: 10.1016/s0065-2660(01)42016-5

[2] Zheng J, Ibrahim S, Petersen F, Yu X. Meta-analysis reveals an association of PTPN22 C1858T with autoimmune diseases, which depends on the localization of the affected tissue. Genes and Immunity. 2012;**13**(8):641-652. DOI: 10.1038/gene.2012.46

[3] Tizaoui K, Kim SH, Jeong GH, et al. Association of PTPN22 1858C/T polymorphism with autoimmune diseases: A systematic review and Bayesian approach. Journal of Clinical Medicine. 2019;**8**(3):347. Published 12 March 2019. DOI: 10.3390/jcm8030347

[4] Cohen S, Dadi H, Shaoul E, Sharfe N, Roifman CM. Cloning and characterization of a lymphoid-specific, inducible human protein tyrosine phosphatase, Lyp. Blood. 1999;**93**:2013-2024

[5] Vang T, Congia M, Macis MD, et al. Autoimmune-associated lymphoid tyrosine phosphatase is a gain-of-function variant. Nature Genetics. 2005;**37**(12):1317-1319. DOI: 10.1038/ng1673

[6] Arechiga AF, Habib T, He Y, et al. Cutting edge: The PTPN22 allelic variant associated with autoimmunity impairs B cell signaling. Journal of Immunology. 2009;**182**:3343-3347

[7] Bottini N, Musumeci L, Alonso A, et al. A functional variant of lymphoid tyrosine phosphatase is associated with type I diabetes. Nature Genetics. 2004;**36**(4):337-338. DOI: 10.1038/ng1323

[8] Bottini N, Vang T, Cucca F, Mustelin T. Role of PTPN22 in type 1 diabetes and other autoimmune diseases. Seminars in Immunology. 2006;**18**:207-213

[9] Singh SP, Wal P, Wal A, Srivastava V, Tiwari R, Sharma RD. Understanding autoimmune disease: An update review. International Journal of Pharmaceutical Technology and Biotechnology. 2016;**3**(3):51-65

[10] Ortonne JP. Recent developments in the understanding of pathogenesis of psoriasis. The British Journal of Dermatology. 1999;**140**(Suppl 54):1-7

[11] Kukreja A, Maclaren NK. Autoimmunity and diabetes. The Journal of Clinical Endocrinology and Metabolism. 1999;**84**:4371-4378

[12] Gregersen PK. Genetic analysis of rheumatic diseases. In: Kelley WN, Harris ED Jr, Ruddy S, Sledge CN, editors. Textbook of Rheumatology. 5th ed. Vol. 1. Philadelphia: W.B. Saunders; 1997. pp. 209-211

[13] Encinas JA, Kuchroo VK. Mapping and identification of autoimmunity genes. Current Opinion in Immunology. 2000;**12**:691-697

[14] Becker KG. Comparative genetics of type I diabetes and autoimmune disease: Common loci, common pathways? Diabetes. 1999;**48**:1353-1358

[15] Sehgal VN, Srivastava G. Vitiligo: Compendium of clinico-epidemiological features. Indian Journal of Dermatology, Venereology and Leprology. 2007;**73**(3):149-156

[16] Guerra L, Dellambra E, Brescia S, Raskovic D. Vitiligo: pathogenetic hypotheses and targets for current therapies. Current Drug Metabolism. 2010;**11**(5):451-467

[17] Krüger C, Schallreuter KU. A review of the worldwide prevalence of vitiligo

in children/adolescents and adults. International Journal of Dermatology. 2012;**51**(10):1206-1212

[18] Jin Y, Bennett DC, Amadi-Myers A, Holland P, Riccardi SL, Gowan K, et al. Vitiligo-associated multiple autoimmune disease is not associated with genetic variation in AIRE. Pigment Cell Research. 2007;**20**(5):402-404

[19] van Geel N, Speeckaert M, Brochez L, Lambert J, Speeckaert R. Clinical profile of generalized vitiligo patients with associated autoimmune/autoinflammatory diseases. Journal of the European Academy of Dermatology and Venereology. 2014;**28**(6):741-746

[20] Garcia-Melendez ME, Salinas-Santander M, Sanchez-Dominguez C, Gonzalez-Cardenas H, Cerda-Flores RM, Ocampo-Candiani J, et al. Protein tyrosine phosphatase PTPN22 + 1858C/T polymorphism is associated with active vitiligo. Experimental and Therapeutic Medicine. 2014;**8**(5):1433-1437

[21] Spritz RA. The genetics of generalized vitiligo and associated autoimmune diseases. Pigment Cell Research. 2007;**20**:271-278

[22] Pehlivan S, Ozkinay F, Alper S, Onay H, Yuksel E, Pehlivan M, et al. Association between IL4 (-590), ACE (I)/(D), CCR5 (Delta32), CTLA4 (+49) and IL1-RN (VNTR in intron 2) gene polymorphisms and vitiligo. European Journal of Dermatology. 2009;**19**(2):126-128

[23] Zamani M, Tabatabaiefar MA, Mosayyebi S, Mashaghi A, Mansouri P. Possible association of the CD4 gene polymorphism with vitiligo in an Iranian population. Clinical and Experimental Dermatology. 2010;**35**(5):521-524

[24] Ochoa-Ramírez LA, Becerra-Loaiza DS, Díaz-Camacho SP, Muñoz-Estrada VF, Ríos-Burgueño ER, Prado-Montes de Oca E, et al. Association of human beta-defensin 1 gene polymorphisms with nonsegmental vitiligo. Clinical and Experimental Dermatology. 2019;**44**(3):277-282. DOI: 10.1111/ced.13697

[25] Rajendiran KS, Rajappa M, Chandrashekar L, Thappa DM. Association of PTPN22 gene polymorphism with non-segmental vitiligoin South Indian Tamils. Postepy Dermatologii I Alergologii. 2018;**35**(3):280-285

[26] Song GG, Kim JH, Lee YH. The CTLA-4 +49 A/G, CT60 A/G and PTPN22 1858 C/T polymorphisms and susceptibility to vitiligo: a meta-analysis. Molecular Biology Reports. 2013;**40**(4):2985-2993

[27] Akbas H, Dertlioglu SB, Dilmec F, Atay AE. Lack of association between PTPN22 Gene +1858 C>T polymorphism and susceptibility to generalized vitiligo in a Turkish population. Annals of Dermatology. 2014;**26**(1):88-91

[28] Agarwal S, Changotra H. Association of protein tyrosine phosphatase, non-receptor type 22 +1858C→T polymorphism and susceptibility to vitiligo: Systematic review and meta-analysis. Indian Journal of Dermatology, Venereology and Leprology. 2017;**83**(2):183-189

[29] Cantón I, Akhtar S, Gavalas NG, Gawkrodger DJ, Blomhoff A, Watson PF, et al. A single-nucleotide polymorphism in the gene encoding lymphoid protein tyrosine phosphatase (PTPN22) confers susceptibility to generalised vitiligo. Genes and Immunity. 2005;**6**:584-587

[30] Laberge GS, Birlea SA, Fain PR, Spritz RA. The PTPN22 – 1858C>T (R620W) functional polymorphism is associated with generalized vitiligo in the Romanian population. Pigment Cell

& Melanoma Research. 2008;**21**: 206-208

[31] Jin Y, Birlea SA, Fain PR, Gowan K, Riccardi SL, Holland PJ, et al. Variant of TYR and autoimmunity susceptibility loci in generalized vitiligo. The New England Journal of Medicine. 2010; **362**(18):1686-1697

[32] Laddha NC, Dwivedi M, Shajil EM, Prajapati H, Marfatia YS, Begum R. Association of PTPN22 1858C/T polymorphism with vitiligo susceptibility in Gujarat population. Journal of Dermatological Science. 2008;**49**:260-262

[33] Alkhateeb A, Qarqaz F, Al-Sabah J, Al Rashaideh T. Clinical characteristics and PTPN22 1858C/T variant analysis in Jordanian Arab vitiligo patients. Molecular Diagnosis & Therapy. 2010; **14**:179-184

[34] Elmongy NN, Abu Khalil RE. PTPN22 gene polymorphism in Egyptian females with non-segmental vitiligo. Comparative Clinical Pathology. 2013;**22**(5):961-964

[35] Galán-Gutiérrez M, Rodríguez-Bujaldón A, Moreno-Giménez JC. Update on the treatment of alopecia areata. Actas Dermo-Sifiliográficas. 2009;**100**:266-276. (In Spanish)

[36] Hordinsky MK. Overview of alopecia areata. The Journal of Investigative Dermatology. Symposium Proceedings. 2013;**16**(1):S13-S15. DOI: 10.1038/jidsymp.2013.4

[37] Alzolibani AA. Epidemiologic and genetic characteristics of alopecia areata (part 1). Acta Dermatovenerologica Alpina, Panonica, et Adriatica. 2011;**20**: 191-198

[38] Kemp EH, McDonagh AJ, Wengraf DA, et al. The non-synonymous C1858T substitution in the PTPN22 gene is associated with susceptibility to the severe forms of alopecia areata. Human Immunology. 2006;**67**(7):535-539. DOI: 10.1016/j.humimm.2006.04.006

[39] Betz RC, König K, Flaquer A, et al. The R620W polymorphism in PTPN22 confers general susceptibility for the development of alopecia areata. The British Journal of Dermatology. 2008; **158**(2):389-391. DOI: 10.1111/j.1365-2133.2007.08312.x

[40] El-Zawahry BM, Azzam OA, Zaki NS, Abdel-Raheem HM, Bassiouny DA, Khorshied MM. PTPN22 gene polymorphism in Egyptian alopecia areata patients and its impact on response to diphencyprone immunotherapy. Gene. 2013;**523**(2): 147-151. DOI: 10.1016/j.gene.2013.03.070

[41] Salinas-Santander M, Sánchez-Domínguez C, Cantú-Salinas C, et al. Association between PTPN22 C1858T polymorphism and alopecia areata risk. Experimental and Therapeutic Medicine. 2015;**10**(5):1953-1958. DOI: 10.3892/etm.2015.2728

[42] Bhanusali DG, Sachdev A, Olson MA, Gerlach JA, Sinha AA. PTPN22 profile indicates a novel risk group in Alopecia areata. Human Immunology. 2014;**75**(1):81-87. DOI: 10.1016/j.humimm.2013.09.003

[43] Lei ZX, Chen WJ, Liang JQ, et al. The association between rs2476601 polymorphism in PTPN22 gene and risk of alopecia areata: A meta-analysis of case-control studies. Medicine (Baltimore). 2019;**98**(20):e15448. DOI: 10.1097/MD.0000000000015448

[44] Moravvej H, Tabatabaei-Panah PS, Abgoon R, et al. Genetic variant association of PTPN22, CTLA4, IL2RA, as well as HLA frequencies in susceptibility to alopecia areata. Immunological Investigations. 2018;

47(7):666-679. DOI: 10.1080/08820139.2018.1480032

[45] Icen M, Crowson CS, McEvoy MT, Dann FJ, Gabriel SE, Maradit KH. Trends in incidence of adult-onset psoriasis over three decades: a population-based study. Journal of the American Academy of Dermatology. 2009;**60**(3):394-401. DOI: 10.1016/j.jaad.2008.10.062

[46] Dogra S, Yadav S. Psoriasis in India: Prevalence and pattern. Indian Journal of Dermatology, Venereology and Leprology. 2010;**76**(6):595-601. DOI: 10.4103/0378-6323.72443

[47] Ding X, Wang T, Shen Y, et al. Prevalence of psoriasis in China: A population-based study in six cities. European Journal of Dermatology. 2012; **22**(5):663-667. DOI: 10.1684/ejd.2012.1802

[48] Choon SE, Lai NM, Mohammad NA, Nanu NM, Tey KE, Chew SF. Clinical profile, morbidity, and outcome of adult-onset generalized pustular psoriasis: Analysis of 102 cases seen in a tertiary hospital in Johor, Malaysia. International Journal of Dermatology. 2014;**53**(6):676-684. DOI: 10.1111/ijd.12070

[49] Loo CH, Chan YC, Lee KQ, Tharmalingam P, Tan WC. Clinical profile, morbidity and outcome of adult patients with psoriasis at a district hospital in Northern Malaysia. The Medical Journal of Malaysia. 2015;**70**(3):177-181

[50] Al Harthi F, Huraib GB, Zouman A, Arfin M, Tariq M, Al-Asmari A. Apolipoprotein E gene polymorphism and serum lipid profile in Saudi patients with psoriasis. Disease Markers. 2014; **2014**:239645. DOI: 10.1155/2014/239645

[51] Elder JT. Genome-wide association scan yields new insights into the immunopathogenesis of psoriasis. Genes and Immunity. 2009;**10**(3):201-209. DOI: 10.1038/gene.2009.11

[52] Elder JT, Bruce AT, Gudjonsson JE, et al. Molecular dissection of psoriasis: integrating genetics and biology. The Journal of Investigative Dermatology. 2010;**130**(5):1213-1226. DOI: 10.1038/jid.2009.319

[53] Scarpa R, Altomare G, Marchesoni A, Balato N, Matucci Cerinic M, Lotti T, et al. Psoriatic disease: Concepts and implications. Journal of the European Academy of Dermatology and Venereology. 2010; **24**(6):627-630. DOI: 10.1111/j.1468-3083.2010.03574.x

[54] Li Y, Chang M, Schrodi SJ, et al. The 5q31 variants associated with psoriasis and Crohn's disease are distinct. Human Molecular Genetics. 2008;**17**(19):2978-2985. DOI: 10.1093/hmg/ddn196

[55] Li Y, Liao W, Chang M, et al. Further genetic evidence for three psoriasis-risk genes: ADAM33, CDKAL1, and PTPN22. The Journal of Investigative Dermatology. 2009; **129**(3):629-634. DOI: 10.1038/jid.2008.297

[56] Chen YF, Chang JS. PTPN22 C1858T and the risk of psoriasis: A meta-analysis. Molecular Biology Reports. 2012;**39**(8):7861-7870. DOI: 10.1007/s11033-012-1630-z

[57] Hüffmeier U, Steffens M, Burkhardt H, et al. Evidence for susceptibility determinant(s) to psoriasis vulgaris in or near PTPN22 in German patients. Journal of Medical Genetics. 2006;**43**(6):517-522. DOI: 10.1136/jmg.2005.037515

[58] Smith RL, Warren RB, Eyre S, Ke X, Young HS, Allen M, et al. Polymorphisms in the PTPN22 region are associated with psoriasis of early onset. The British Journal of

Dermatology. 2008;**158**(5):962-968. DOI: 10.1111/j.1365-2133.2008.08482.x

[59] Nistor I, Nair RP, Stuart P, et al. Protein tyrosine phosphatase gene PTPN22 polymorphism in psoriasis: Lack of evidence for association. The Journal of Investigative Dermatology. 2005;**125**(2):395-396. DOI: 10.1111/j.0022-202X.2005.23802.x

[60] Zervou MI, Castro-Giner F, Sidiropoulos P, Boumpas DT, Tosca AD, Krueger-Krasagakis S. The protein tyrosine phosphatase, non-receptor type 22 R620W polymorphism does not confer susceptibility to psoriasis in the genetic homogeneous population of Crete. Genetic Testing and Molecular Biomarkers. 2010;**14**(1):107-111

[61] Butt C, Peddle L, Greenwood C, Hamilton S, Gladman D, Rahman P. Association of functional variants of PTPN22 and tp53 in psoriatic arthritis: a case-control study. Arthritis Research & Therapy. 2006;**8**(1):R27. DOI: 10.1186/ar1880

[62] Juneblad K, Johansson M, Rantapää-Dahlqvist S, Alenius GM. Association between the PTPN22 +1858 C/T polymorphism and psoriatic arthritis. Arthritis Research and Therapy. 2011; **13**(2):R45. Published Mar 16, 2011. DOI: 10.1186/ar3284

[63] Bowes J, Loehr S, Budu-Aggrey A, et al. PTPN22 is associated with susceptibility to psoriatic arthritis but not psoriasis: Evidence for a further PsA-specific risk locus. Annals of the Rheumatic Diseases. 2015;**74**(10): 1882-1885. DOI: 10.1136/annrheumdis-2014-207187

[64] Budu-Aggrey A, Bowes J, Barton A. Identifying a novel locus for psoriatic arthritis. Rheumatology (Oxford, England). 2016;**55**(1):25-32. DOI: 10.1093/rheumatology/kev273

[65] Hinks A, Barton A, John S, et al. Association between the PTPN22 gene and rheumatoid arthritis and juvenile idiopathic arthritis in a UK population: Further support that PTPN22 is an autoimmunity gene. Arthritis and Rheumatism. 2005;**52**(6):1694-1699. DOI: 10.1002/art.21049

[66] Hüffmeier U, Reis A, Steffens M, et al. Male restricted genetic association of variant R620W in PTPN22 with psoriatic arthritis. The Journal of Investigative Dermatology. 2006; **126**(4):932-935. DOI: 10.1038/sj.jid.5700179

[67] Kaalla MJ, Broadaway KA, Rohani-Pichavant M, et al. Meta-analysis confirms association between TNFA-G238A variant and JIA, and between PTPN22-C1858T variant and oligoarticular, RF-polyarticular and RF-positive polyarticular JIA. Pediatric Rheumatology Online Journal. 2013; **11**(1):40. Published Oct 25, 2013. DOI: 10.1186/1546-0096-11-40

[68] Hinks A, Eyre S, Ke X, Barton A, Martin P, Flynn E, et al. Overlap of disease susceptibility loci for rheumatoid arthritis and juvenile idiopathic arthritis. Annals of the Rheumatic Diseases. 2010;**69**(6): 1049-1053. DOI: 10.1136/ard.2009.110650

[69] Thompson SD, Sudman M, Ramos PS, Marion MC, Ryan M, Tsoras M, et al. The susceptibility loci juvenile idiopathic arthritis shares with other autoimmune diseases extend to PTPN2, COG6, and ANGPT1. Arthritis and Rheumatism. 2010;**62**(11):3265-3276. DOI: 10.1002/art.27688

[70] Ellis JA, Chavez RA, Pezic A, Ponsonby AL, Akikusa JD, Allen RC, et al. Independent replication analysis of genetic loci with previous evidence of association with juvenile idiopathic arthritis. Pediatric Rheumatology Online Journal. 2013;**11**(1):12. DOI: 10.1186/1546-0096-11-12

[71] Chiaroni-Clarke RC, Li YR, Munro JE, et al. The association of PTPN22 rs2476601 with juvenile idiopathic arthritis is specific to females. Genes and Immunity. 2015;**16**(7): 495-498. DOI: 10.1038/gene.2015. 32

[72] Cinek O, Hradsky O, Ahmedov G, Slavcev A, Kolouskova S, Kulich M, et al. No independent role of the −1123 G>C and +2740 A>G variants in the association of PTPN22 with type 1 diabetes and juvenile idiopathic arthritis in two Caucasian populations. Diabetes Research and Clinical Practice. 2007; **76**(2):297-303. DOI: 10.1016/j. diabres.2006.09.009

[73] Goulielmos GN, Chiaroni-Clarke RC, Dimopoulou DG, et al. Association of juvenile idiopathic arthritis with PTPN22 rs2476601 is specific to females in a Greek population. Pediatric Rheumatology Online Journal. 2016; **14**(1):25. DOI: 10.1186/s12969-016-0087-3

[74] Viken MK, Amundsen SS, Kvien TK, Boberg KM, Gilboe IM, Lilleby V, et al. Association analysis of the 1858C>T polymorphism in the PTPN22 gene in juvenile idiopathic arthritis and other autoimmune diseases. Genes and Immunity. 2005; **6**(3):271-273. DOI: 10.1038/sj. gene.6364178

[75] Soliman YA, Hashaad NI, Emam SM, Mohamed RR. Role of PTPN22 1858 C/T polymorphisms in juvenile idiopathic arthritis in Egyptian patients. The Egyptian Journal of Immunology. 2017;**24**(1):95-104

[76] Lee YH, Bae SC, Song GG. The association between the functional PTPN22 1858 C/T and MIF −173 C/G polymorphisms and juvenile idiopathic arthritis: a meta-analysis. Inflammation Research. 2012;**61**(5):411-415. DOI: 10.1007/s00011-012-0447-5

[77] DI Y, Zhong S, Wu L, Li Y, Sun N. The association between PTPN22 genetic polymorphism and juvenile idiopathic arthritis (JIA) susceptibility: An updated meta-analysis. Iranian Journal of Public Health. 2015;**44**(9): 1169-1175

[78] Seldin MF, Shigeta R, Laiho K, Li H, Saila H, Savolainen A, et al. Finnish case-control and family studies support PTPN22 R620W polymorphism as a risk factor in rheumatoid arthritis, but suggest only minimal or no effect in juvenile idiopathic arthritis. Genes and Immunity. 2005;**6**(8):720-722

[79] Pazar B, Gergely P Jr, Nagy ZB, Gombos T, Pozsonyi E, Rajczy K, et al. Role of HLA-DRB1 and PTPN22 genes in susceptibility to juvenile idiopathic arthritis in Hungarian patients. Clinical and Experimental Rheumatology. 2008; **26**(6):1146-1152

[80] Chaudhari K, Rizvi S, Syed BA. Rheumatoid arthritis: current and future trends. Nature Reviews Drug Discovery. 2016;**15**(5):305-306. DOI: 10.1038/ nrd.2016.21

[81] Angelotti F, Parma A, Cafaro G, Capecchi R, Alunno A, Puxeddu I. One year in review 2017: Pathogenesis of rheumatoid arthritis. Clinical and Experimental Rheumatology. 2017; **35**(3):368-378

[82] McInnes IB, Schett G. The pathogenesis of rheumatoid arthritis. The New England Journal of Medicine. 2011;**365**(23):2205-2219. DOI: 10.1056/ NEJMra1004965

[83] Shaik NA, Banaganapalli B. Computational molecular phenotypic analysis of PTPN22 (W620R), IL6R (D358A), and TYK2 (P1104A) gene mutations of rheumatoid arthritis. Frontiers in Genetics. 2019;**10**:168. DOI: 10.3389/fgene.2019.00168

[84] Abbasi Z, Kazemi Nezhad SR, Pourmahdi-Broojeni M, Rajaei E. Association of PTPN22 rs2476601

polymorphism with rheumatoid arthritis and celiac disease in Khuzestan province. Southwestern Iran. Iranian Biomedical Journal. 2017;**21**(1):61-66. DOI: 10.6091/.21.1.61

[85] Fodil M, Benzaoui A, Zemani-Fodil F, et al. Association of PTPN22 (rs2476601) and STAT4 (rs7574865) polymorphisms with rheumatoid arthritis in the Western Algerian population. Acta Reumatológica Portuguesa. 2015;**40**(1):56-62

[86] Gomez LM, Anaya JM, Gonzalez CI, Pineda-Tamayo R, Otero W, Arango A, et al. PTPN22 C1858T polymorphism in Colombian patients with autoimmune diseases. Genes and Immunity. 2005;**6**: 628-631. DOI: 10.1038/sj.gene.6364261

[87] Ramirez M, Quintana G, Diaz-Gallo LM, et al. The PTPN22 C1858T variant as a risk factor for rheumatoid arthritis and systemic lupus erythematosus but not for systemic sclerosis in the Colombian population. Clinical and Experimental Rheumatology. 2012; **30**(4):520-524

[88] Salama A, Elshazli R, Elsaid A, Settin A. Protein tyrosine phosphatase non-receptor type 22 (PTPN22) +1858 C>T gene polymorphism in Egyptian cases with rheumatoid arthritis. Cellular Immunology. 2014;**290**(1):62-65. DOI: 10.1016/j.cellimm.2014.05.003

[89] Raslan HM, Attia HR, Salama I, et al. Association of PTPN22 1858C→T polymorphism, HLA-DRB1 shared epitope and autoantibodies with rheumatoid arthritis. Rheumatology International. 2016;**36**(8):1167-1175. DOI: 10.1007/s00296-016-3511-6

[90] Hegab MM, Abdelwahab AF, El-Sayed Yousef AM, et al. CD28 and PTPN22 are associated with susceptibility to rheumatoid arthritis in Egyptians. Human Immunology. 2016; **77**(6):522-526. DOI: 10.1016/j.humimm.2016.04.018

[91] Hashemi M, Atabaki M, Daneshvar H, Zakeri Z, Eskandari-Nasab E. Association of PTPN22 rs2476601 and EGFR rs17337023 Gene polymorphisms and rheumatoid arthritis in Zahedan, Southeast Iran. International Journal of Immunogenetics. 2013;**40**(4):299-305

[92] Totaro MC, Tolusso B, Napolioni V, et al. PTPN22 1858C>T polymorphism distribution in Europe and association with rheumatoid arthritis: Case-control study and meta-analysis. PLoS One. 2011;**6**(9):e24292. DOI: 10.1371/journal.pone.0024292

[93] Torres-Carrillo NM, Ruiz-Noa Y, Martínez-Bonilla GE, et al. The +1858C/T PTPN22 gene polymorphism confers genetic susceptibility to rheumatoid arthritis in Mexican population from the Western Mexico. Immunology Letters. 2012;**147**(1-2):41-46. DOI: 10.1016/j.imlet.2012.05.007

[94] Rincón JF, Cano DL, Morales SJ, Jiménez ML, Cobos RE, Bello JR. The functional PTPN22 C1858T polymorphism confers risk for rheumatoid arthritis in patients from Central Mexico. Clinical Rheumatology. 2016;**35**(6):1457-1462. DOI: 10.1007/s10067-016-3223-z

[95] Ruiz-Noa Y, Padilla-Gutiérrez JR, Hernández-Bello J, et al. Association of *PTPN22* haplotypes (−1123G>C/+1858C>T) with rheumatoid arthritis in Western Mexican population. International Journal of Genomics. 2017; **2017**:8753498. DOI: 10.1155/2017/8753498

[96] Orozco G, Sánchez E, González-Gay MA, et al. Association of a functional single-nucleotide polymorphism of PTPN22, encoding lymphoid protein phosphatase, with rheumatoid arthritis and systemic lupus erythematosus. Arthritis and Rheumatism. 2005;**52**(1):219-224. DOI: 10.1002/art.20771

[97] Ates A, Karaaslan Y, Karatayli E, et al. Association of the PTPN22 gene polymorphism with autoantibody positivity in Turkish rheumatoid arthritis patients. Tissue Antigens. 2011; **78**(1):56-59. DOI: 10.1111/j.1399-0039.2011.01675.x

[98] Li Q, Lin KQ, Li Q, et al. Association of polymorphisms of PTPN22 and PADI4 genes with rheumatoid arthritis in Yunnan. Zhonghua Yi Xue Yi Chuan Xue Za Zhi. 2013;**30**(1):111-115. DOI: 10.3760/cma.j.issn.1003-9406.2013.01.027

[99] Tang L, Wang Y, Zheng S, Bao M, Zhang Q, Li J. PTPN22 polymorphisms, but not R620W, were associated with the genetic susceptibility of systemic lupus erythematosus and rheumatoid arthritis in a Chinese Han population. Human Immunology. 2016;**77**(8): 692-698. DOI: 10.1016/j.humimm.2016.04.021

[100] El-Lebedy D, Raslan H, Ibrahim A, Ashmawy I, El-Aziz SA, Mohammed AM. Association of STAT4 rs7574865 and PTPN22 rs2476601 polymorphisms with rheumatoid arthritis and non-systemically reacting antibodies in Egyptian patients. Clinical Rheumatology. 2017;**36**(9):1981-1987. DOI: 10.1007/s10067-017-3632-7

[101] Ahmadloo S, Taghizadeh M, Akhiani M, Salimzadeh A, Keramatipour M. Single Nucleotide Polymorphism rs 2476601 of PTPN22 Gene and Susceptibility to Rheumatoid Arthritis in Iranian Population. Iranian Journal of Allergy, Asthma, and Immunology. 2015;**14**(4):437-442

[102] Song GG, Bae SC, Kim JH, Lee YH. The PTPN22 C1858T polymorphism and rheumatoid arthritis: A meta-analysis. Rheumatology International. 2013; **33**(8):1991-1999. DOI: 10.1007/s00296-013-2679-2

[103] Nabi G, Akhter N, Wahid M, et al. Meta-analysis reveals PTPN22 1858C/T polymorphism confers susceptibility to rheumatoid arthritis in Caucasian but not in Asian population. Autoimmunity. 2016;**49**(3):197-210. DOI: 10.3109/08916934.2015.1134514

[104] Elshazli R, Settin A. Association of PTPN22 rs2476601 and STAT4 rs7574865 polymorphisms with rheumatoid arthritis: A meta-analysis update. Immunobiology. 2015;**220**(8): 1012-1024. DOI: 10.1016/j.imbio.2015.04.003

[105] Nong LM, Ren KW, Xu NW, Zhou D. 1858 C/T polymorphism of the protein tyrosine phosphatase nonreceptor 22 gene and rheumatoid arthritis risk in Europeans: A meta-analysis. Archives of Medical Research. 2011;**42**(8):698-702. DOI: 10.1016/j.arcmed.2011.12.001

[106] Plant D, Flynn E, Mbarek H, et al. Investigation of potential non-HLA rheumatoid arthritis susceptibility loci in a European cohort increases the evidence for nine markers. Annals of the Rheumatic Diseases. 2010;**69**(8): 1548-1553. DOI: 10.1136/ard.2009.121020

[107] Lee YH, Rho YH, Choi SJ, et al. The PTPN22 C1858T functional polymorphism and autoimmune diseases—A meta-analysis. Rheumatology (Oxford, England). 2007;**46**(1):49-56. DOI: 10.1093/rheumatology/kel170

[108] Jiang Y, Zhang R, Zheng J, et al. Meta-analysis of 125 rheumatoid arthritis-related single nucleotide polymorphisms studied in the past two decades. PLoS One. 2012;**7**(12):e51571. DOI: 10.1371/journal.pone.0051571

[109] Meza-Meza MR, Vizmanos-Lamotte B, Muñoz-Valle JF, et al. Relationship of excess weight with clinical activity and dietary intake deficiencies in systemic lupus erythematosus patients. Nutrients.

2019;**11**(11):E2683. Published Nov 6, 2019. DOI: 10.3390/nu11112683

[110] Carter EE, Barr SG, Clarke AE. The global burden of SLE: Prevalence, health disparities and socioeconomic impact. Nature Reviews Rheumatology. 2016; **12**(10):605-620. DOI: 10.1038/nrrheum.2016.137

[111] Mak A, Tay SH. Environmental factors, toxicants and systemic lupus erythematosus. International Journal of Molecular Sciences. 2014;**15**(9): 16043-16056. Published Sep 11, 2014. DOI: 10.3390/ijms150916043

[112] Kwon YC, Chun S, Kim K, Mak A. Update on the genetics of systemic lupus erythematosus: genome-wide association studies and beyond. Cells. 2019;**8**(10):1180. Published Sep 30, 2019. DOI: 10.3390/cells8101180

[113] Buniello A, MacArthur JAL, Cerezo M, et al. The NHGRI-EBI GWAS Catalog of published genome-wide association studies, targeted arrays and summary statistics 2019. Nucleic Acids Research. 2019;**47**(D1):D1005-D1012. DOI: 10.1093/nar/gky1120

[114] Morris DL, Sheng Y, Zhang Y, et al. Genome-wide association meta-analysis in Chinese and European individuals identifies ten new loci associated with systemic lupus erythematosus. Nature Genetics. 2016;**48**(8):940-946. DOI: 10.1038/ng.3603

[115] Sun C, Molineros JE, Looger LL, et al. High-density genotyping of immune-related loci identifies new SLE risk variants in individuals with Asian ancestry. Nature Genetics. 2016;**48**(3):323-330. DOI: 10.1038/ng.3496

[116] Kyogoku C, Langefeld CD, Ortmann WA, et al. Genetic association of the R620W polymorphism of protein tyrosine phosphatase PTPN22 with human SLE. American Journal of Human Genetics. 2004;**75**(3):504-507. DOI: 10.1086/423790

[117] Kaufman KM, Kelly JA, Herring BJ, et al. Evaluation of the genetic association of the PTPN22 R620W polymorphism in familial and sporadic systemic lupus erythematosus. Arthritis and Rheumatism. 2006;**54**(8): 2533-2540. DOI: 10.1002/art.21963

[118] Namjou B, Kim-Howard X, Sun C, et al. PTPN22 association in systemic lupus erythematosus (SLE) with respect to individual ancestry and clinical sub-phenotypes. PLoS One. 2013;**8**(8): e69404. DOI: 10.1371/journal.pone.0069404

[119] Eliopoulos E, Zervou MI, Andreou A, et al. Association of the PTPN22 R620W polymorphism with increased risk for SLE in the genetically homogeneous population of Crete. Lupus. 2011;**20**(5):501-506. DOI: 10.1177/0961203310392423

[120] Reddy MV, Johansson M, Sturfelt G, et al. The R620W C/T polymorphism of the gene PTPN22 is associated with SLE independently of the association of PDCD1. Genes and Immunity. 2005;**6**(8):658-662. DOI: 10.1038/sj.gene.6364252

[121] Piotrowski P, Lianeri M, Wudarski M, Lacki JK, Jagodziński PP. Contribution of the R620W polymorphism of protein tyrosine phosphatase non-receptor 22 to systemic lupus erythematosus in Poland. Clinical and Experimental Rheumatology. 2008;**26**(6): 1099-1102

[122] Ostanek L, Ostanek-Pańka M, Bobrowska-Snarska D, et al. PTPN22 1858C>T gene polymorphism in patients with SLE: Association with serological and clinical results. Molecular Biology Reports. 2014;**41**(9): 6195-6200. DOI: 10.1007/s11033-014-3498-6

[123] Moez P, Soliman E. Association of PTPN22 gene polymorphism and systemic lupus erythematosus in a cohort of Egyptian patients: Impact on clinical and laboratory results. Rheumatology International. 2012; **32**(9):2753-2758. DOI: 10.1007/s00296-011-2063-z

[124] Elghzaly AA, Metwally SS, El-Chennawi FA, et al. IRF5, PTPN22, CD28, IL2RA, KIF5A, BLK and TNFAIP3 genes polymorphisms and lupus susceptibility in a cohort from the Egypt Delta; relation to other ethnic groups. Human Immunology. 2015; **76**(7):525-531. DOI: 10.1016/j.humimm.2015.06.001

[125] Lea WW, Lee YH. The association between the PTPN22 C1858T polymorphism and systemic lupus erythematosus: A meta-analysis update. Lupus. 2011;**20**(1):51-57. DOI: 10.1177/0961203310381774

[126] Shi L, Wei Y, Xun W, Han D. Meta-analysis of the correlation between PTPN22 gene polymorphisms and susceptibility to systemic lupus erythematosus. Asia-Pacific Journal of Public Health. 2013;**25**(4 Suppl):22S-29S. DOI: 10.1177/1010539513496268

[127] de Lima SC, Adelino JE, Crovella S, de Azevedo Silva J, Sandrin-Garcia P. PTPN22 1858C>T polymorphism and susceptibility to systemic lupus erythematosus: a meta-analysis update. Autoimmunity. 2017;**50**(7):428-434. DOI: 10.1080/08916934.2017.1385774

[128] Hu LY, Cheng Z, Zhang B, et al. Associations between PTPN22 and TLR9 polymorphisms and systemic lupus erythematosus: A comprehensive meta-analysis. Archives of Dermatological Research. 2017;**309**(6): 461-477. DOI: 10.1007/s00403-017-1745-0

[129] Peng XB, Ou LN. Correlation between PTPN22 gene polymorphism and systemic lupus erythematosus in Chinese Han patients. Nan Fang Yi Ke Da Xue Xue Bao. 2010;**30**(10): 2390-2391

[130] Machado-Contreras JR, Muñoz-Valle JF, Cruz A, Salazar-Camarena DC, Marín-Rosales M, Palafox-Sánchez CA. Distribution of PTPN22 polymorphisms in SLE from western Mexico: correlation with mRNA expression and disease activity. Clinical and Experimental Medicine. 2016;**16**(3): 399-406. DOI: 10.1007/s10238-015-0359-0

[131] Zervou MI, Vazgiourakis VM, Yilmaz N, et al. TRAF1/C5, eNOS, C1q, but not STAT4 and PTPN22 gene polymorphisms are associated with genetic susceptibility to systemic lupus erythematosus in Turkey. Human Immunology. 2011;**72**(12): 1210-1213. DOI: 10.1016/j.humimm.2011.09.003

[132] Aksoy R, Duman T, Keskin O, Düzgün N. No association of PTPN22 R620W gene polymorphism with rheumatic heart disease and systemic lupus erythematosus. Molecular Biology Reports. 2011;**38**(8):5393-5396. DOI: 10.1007/s11033-011-0692-7

[133] Hamza RT, Awwad KS, Temsah KA, Hamed AI. R620W polymorphism of protein tyrosine phosphatase PTPN22 in Egyptian children and adolescents with systemic lupus erythematosus: relation to thyroid autoimmunity. International Journal of Adolescent Medicine and Health. 2013; **25**(2):143-149. DOI: 10.1515/ijamh-2013-0022

[134] Baca V, Velázquez-Cruz R, Salas-Martínez G, Espinosa-Rosales F, Saldaña-Alvarez Y, Orozco L. Association analysis of the PTPN22 gene in childhood-onset systemic lupus erythematosus in Mexican population. Genes and Immunity. 2006;**7**(8): 693-695. DOI: 10.1038/sj.gene.6364350

[135] Antonelli A, Ferrari SM, Corrado A, Di Domenicantonio A, Fallahi P. Autoimmune thyroid disorders. Autoimmunity Reviews 2015; **14**(2):174-180. DOI: 10.1016/j.autrev.2014.10.016

[136] Tomer Y, Davies TF. Searching for the autoimmune thyroid disease susceptibility genes: from gene mapping to gene function. Endocrine Reviews. 2003;**24**(5):694-717. DOI: 10.1210/er.2002-0030

[137] Tomer Y, Ban Y, Concepcion E, et al. Common and unique susceptibility loci in Graves and Hashimoto diseases: results of whole-genome screening in a data set of 102 multiplex families. American Journal of Human Genetics. 2003;**73**(4):736-747. DOI: 10.1086/378588

[138] Dultz G, Matheis N, Dittmar M, Röhrig B, Bender K, Kahaly GJ. The protein tyrosine phosphatase non-receptor type 22 C1858T polymorphism is a joint susceptibility locus for immune thyroiditis and autoimmune diabetes. Thyroid. 2009;**19**(2):143-148. DOI: 10.1089/thy.2008.0301

[139] Luo L, Cai B, Liu F, Hu X, Wang L. Association of protein tyrosine phosphatase nonreceptor 22 (PTPN22) C1858T gene polymorphism with susceptibility to autoimmune thyroid diseases: A meta-analysis. Endocrine Journal. 2012;**59**(5):439-445. DOI: 10.1507/endocrj.ej11-0381

[140] Heward JM, Brand OJ, Barrett JC, Carr-Smith JD, Franklyn JA, Gough SC. Association of PTPN22 haplotypes with Graves' disease. The Journal of Clinical Endocrinology and Metabolism. 2007; **92**(2):685-690. DOI: 10.1210/jc.2006-2064

[141] Gu LQ, Zhu W, Zhao SX, et al. Clinical associations of the genetic variants of CTLA-4, Tg, TSHR, PTPN22, PTPN12 and FCRL3 in patients with Graves' disease. Clinical Endocrinology. 2010;**72**(2):248-255. DOI: 10.1111/j.1365-2265.2009.03617.x

[142] Zhebrun D, Kudryashova Y, Babenko A, et al. Association of PTPN22 1858T/T genotype with type 1 diabetes, Graves' disease but not with rheumatoid arthritis in Russian population. Aging (Albany, NY). 2011;**3**(4):368-373. DOI: 10.18632/aging.100305

[143] Ban Y, Tozaki T, Taniyama M, et al. Association of the protein tyrosine phosphatase nonreceptor 22 haplotypes with autoimmune thyroid disease in the Japanese population. Thyroid. 2010; **20**(8):893-899. DOI: 10.1089/thy.2010.0104

[144] Ban Y, Tozaki T, Taniyama M, Tomita M, Ban Y. The codon 620 single nucleotide polymorphism of the protein tyrosine phosphatase-22 gene does not contribute to autoimmune thyroid disease susceptibility in the Japanese. Thyroid. 2005;**15**(10):1115-1118. DOI: 10.1089/thy.2005.15.1115

[145] Lee HS, Kang J, Yang S, Kim D, Park Y. Susceptibility influence of a PTPN22 haplotype with thyroid autoimmunity in Koreans. Diabetes/Metabolism Research and Reviews. 2011;**27**(8):878-882. DOI: 10.1002/dmrr.1265

[146] Alkhateeb A, Marzouka NA, Tashtoush R. Variants in PTPN22 and SMOC2 genes and the risk of thyroid disease in the Jordanian Arab population. Endocrine. 2013;**44**(3): 702-709. DOI: 10.1007/s12020-013-9908-z

[147] Krupińska J, Urbanowicz W, Kaczmarczyk M, et al. Association between genetic mutations and the development of autoimmune thyroiditis in patients with chronic hepatitis C treated with interferon alpha. Thyroid Research. 2012;**5**(1):10. DOI: 10.1186/1756-6614-5-10

[148] López-Cano DJ, Cadena-Sandoval D, Beltrán-Ramírez O, et al. The PTPN22 R263Q polymorphism confers protection against systemic lupus erythematosus and rheumatoid arthritis, while PTPN22 R620W confers susceptibility to Graves' disease in a Mexican population. Inflammation Research. 2017;**66**(9):775-781. DOI: 10.1007/s00011-017-1056-0

[149] Wawrusiewicz-Kurylonek N, Koper-Lenkiewicz OM, Gościk J, Myśliwiec J, Pawłowski P, Krętowski AJ. Association of PTPN22 polymorphism and its correlation with Graves' disease susceptibility in Polish adult population-A preliminary study. Molecular Genetics & Genomic Medicine. 2019;**7**(6):e661. DOI: 10.1002/mgg3.661

[150] Skórka A, Bednarczuk T, Bar-Andziak E, Nauman J, Ploski R. Lymphoid tyrosine phosphatase (PTPN22/LYP) variant and Graves' disease in a Polish population: association and gene dose-dependent correlation with age of onset. Clinical Endocrinology. 2005;**62**(6):679-682. DOI: 10.1111/j.1365-2265.2005.02279.x

[151] Velaga MR, Wilson V, Jennings CE, et al. The codon 620 tryptophan allele of the lymphoid tyrosine phosphatase (LYP) gene is a major determinant of Graves' disease. The Journal of Clinical Endocrinology and Metabolism. 2004; **89**(11):5862-5865. DOI: 10.1210/jc.2004-1108

[152] Smyth D, Cooper JD, Collins JE, et al. Replication of an association between the lymphoid tyrosine phosphatase locus (LYP/PTPN22) with type 1 diabetes, and evidence for its role as a general autoimmunity locus. Diabetes. 2004;**53**(11):3020-3023. DOI: 10.2337/diabetes.53.11.3020

[153] Xue L, Pan C, Gu Z, et al. Genetic heterogeneity of susceptibility gene in different ethnic populations: Refining association study of PTPN22 for Graves' disease in a Chinese Han population. PLoS One. 2013;**8**(12):e84514. DOI: 10.1371/journal.pone.0084514

[154] Jurecka-Lubieniecka B, Ploski R, Kula D, et al. Association between age at diagnosis of Graves' disease and variants in genes involved in immune response. PLoS One. 2013;**8**(3):e59349. DOI: 10.1371/journal.pone.0059349

[155] Shehjar F, Afroze D, Misgar RA, Malik SA, Laway BA. PTPN22 1858 C/T exon polymorphism is not associated with graves' disease in Kashmiri population. Indian Journal of Endocrinology and Metabolis. 2018; **22**(4):457-460. DOI: 10.4103/ijem.IJEM_105_18

[156] Jacobson EM, Tomer Y. The genetic basis of thyroid autoimmunity. Thyroid. 2007;**17**(10):949-961. DOI: 10.1089/thy.2007.0153

[157] Gong L, Liu B, Wang J, et al. Novel missense mutation in PTPN22 in a Chinese pedigree with Hashimoto's thyroiditis. BMC Endocrine Disorders. 2018;**18**(1):76. Published Nov 1, 2018. DOI: 10.1186/s12902-018-0305-8

[158] Strober W, Fuss I, Mannon P. The fundamental basis of inflammatory bowel disease. The Journal of Clinical Investigation. 2007;**117**(3):514-521. DOI: 10.1172/JCI30587

[159] Xavier RJ, Podolsky DK. Unravelling the pathogenesis of inflammatory bowel disease. Nature. 2007;**448**(7152):427-434. DOI: 10.1038/nature06005

[160] Kim ES, Kim WH. Inflammatory bowel disease in Korea: Epidemiological, genomic, clinical, and therapeutic characteristics. Gut and Liver. 2010;**4**: 1-14

[161] Waterman M, Xu W, Stempak JM, et al. Distinct and overlapping genetic loci in Crohn's disease and ulcerative

colitis: Correlations with pathogenesis. Inflammatory Bowel Diseases. 2011;**17**: 1936-1942

[162] Al-Meghaiseeb ES, Al-Robayan AA, Al-Otaibi MM, Arfin M, Al-Asmari AK. Association of tumor necrosis factor-α and -β gene polymorphisms in inflammatory bowel disease. Journal of Inflammation Research. 2016;**9**:133-140. DOI: 10.2147/JIR.S101225

[163] Sfar I, Ben Aleya W, Mouelhi L, et al. Lymphoid tyrosine phosphatase R620W variant and inflammatory bowel disease in Tunisia. World Journal of Gastroenterology. 2010;**16**(4): 479-483. DOI: 10.3748/wjg.v16.i4.479

[164] Hedjoudje A, Cheurfa C, Briquez C, Zhang A, Koch S, Vuitton L. rs2476601 polymorphism in *PTPN22* is associated with Crohn's disease but not with ulcerative colitis: A meta-analysis of 16,838 cases and 13,356 controls. Annals of Gastroenterology. 2017;**30**(2): 197-208. DOI: 10.20524/aog.2017.0121

[165] Diaz-Gallo LM, Espino-Paisán L, Fransen K, et al. Differential association of two PTPN22 coding variants with Crohn's disease and ulcerative colitis. Inflammatory Bowel Diseases. 2011; **17**(11):2287-2294. DOI: 10.1002/ibd.21630

[166] Begovich AB, Carlton VE, Honigberg LA, et al. A missense single-nucleotide polymorphism in a gene encoding a protein tyrosine phosphatase (PTPN22) is associated with rheumatoid arthritis. American Journal of Human Genetics. 2004;**75**(2):330-337. DOI: 10.1086/422827

[167] Zaid Y, Senhaji N, Bakhtaoui FZ, et al. The PTPN22 C1858T (R620W) functional polymorphism in inflammatory bowel disease. BMC Research Notes. 2018;**11**(1):783. DOI: 10.1186/s13104-018-3875-7

[168] Morgan AR, Han DY, Huebner C, Lam WJ, Fraser AG, Ferguson LR. PTPN2 but not PTPN22 is associated with Crohn's disease in a New Zealand population. Tissue Antigens. 2010; **76**(2):119-125. DOI: 10.1111/j.1399-0039.2010.01493.x

[169] Hradsky O, Lenicek M, Dusatkova P, et al. Variants of CARD15, TNFA and PTPN22 and susceptibility to Crohn's disease in the Czech population: high frequency of the CARD15 1007fs. Tissue Antigens. 2008;**71**(6):538-547. DOI: 10.1111/j.1399-0039.2008.01047.x

[170] van Oene M, Wintle RF, Liu X, et al. Association of the lymphoid tyrosine phosphatase R620W variant with rheumatoid arthritis, but not Crohn's disease, in Canadian populations. Arthritis and Rheumatism. 2005;**52**(7):1993-1998. DOI: 10.1002/art.21123

[171] De Jager PL, Sawcer S, Waliszewska A, et al. Evaluating the role of the 620W allele of protein tyrosine phosphatase PTPN22 in Crohn's disease and multiple sclerosis. European Journal of Human Genetics. 2006;**14**(3): 317-321. DOI: 10.1038/sj.ejhg.5201548

[172] Prescott NJ, Fisher SA, Onnie C, et al. A general autoimmunity gene (PTPN22) is not associated with inflammatory bowel disease in a British population. Tissue Antigens. 2005; **66**(4):318-320. DOI: 10.1111/j.1399-0039.2005.00494.x

[173] Martín MC, Oliver J, Urcelay E, et al. The functional genetic variation in the PTPN22 gene has a negligible effect on the susceptibility to develop inflammatory bowel disease. Tissue Antigens. 2005;**66**(4):314-317. DOI: 10.1111/j.1399-0039.2005.00428.x

[174] Wagenleiter SE, Klein W, Griga T, Schmiegel W, Epplen JT, Jagiello P. A case-control study of tyrosine phosphatase (PTPN22) confirms the lack of association with Crohn's disease. International Journal of

Immunogenetics. 2005;**32**(5):323-324. DOI: 10.1111/j.1744-313X.2005.00534.x

[175] Latiano A, Palmieri O, Valvano MR, et al. Evaluating the role of the genetic variations of PTPN22, NFKB1, and FcGRIIIA genes in inflammatory bowel disease: A meta-analysis. Inflammatory Bowel Diseases. 2007;**13**(10):1212-1219. DOI: 10.1002/ibd.20185

[176] Guariguata L, Whiting DR, Hambleton I, Beagley J, Linnenkamp U, Shaw JE. Global estimates of diabetes prevalence for 2013 and projections for 2035. Diabetes Research and Clinical Practice. 2014;**103**(2):137-149. DOI: 10.1016/j.diabres.2013.11.002

[177] International Diabetes Federation. IDF Diabetes Atlas. 8th ed. Brussels, Belgium: International Diabetes Federation; 2017. http://www.diabetesa tlas.org

[178] Pei Z, Chen X, Sun C, et al. A novel single nucleotide polymorphism in the protein tyrosine phosphatase N22 gene (PTPN22) is associated with Type 1 diabetes in a Chinese population. Diabetic Medicine. 2014;**31**(2):219-226. DOI: 10.1111/dme.12331

[179] Giza S, Goulas A, Gbandi E, et al. The role of PTPN22 C1858T gene polymorphism in diabetes mellitus type 1: First evaluation in Greek children and adolescents. BioMed Research International. 2013;**721604**:2013. DOI: 10.1155/2013/721604

[180] Baniasadi V, Das SN. No evidence for association of PTPN22 R620W functional variant C1858T with type 1 diabetes in Asian Indians. Journal of Cellular and Molecular Medicine. 2008; **12**(3):1061-1062. DOI: 10.1111/j.1582-4934.2008.00222.x

[181] Almasi S, Aliparasti MR, Yazdchi-Marandi L, et al. Analysis of PTPN22 C1858T gene polymorphism in cases with type 1 diabetes of Azerbaijan, Northwest Iran. Cellular Immunology. 2014;**292**(1-2):14-18. DOI: 10.1016/j.cellimm.2014.08.007

[182] Prezioso G, Comegna L, Di Giulio C, Franchini S, Chiarelli F, Blasetti A. C1858T polymorphism of protein tyrosine phosphatase non-receptor type 22 (PTPN22): An eligible target for prevention of type 1 diabetes?. Expert Review of Clinical Immunology 2017;**13**(3):189-196. DOI: 10.1080/1744666X.2017.1266257

[183] Kawasaki E, Awata T, Ikegami H, et al. Systematic search for single nucleotide polymorphisms in a lymphoid tyrosine phosphatase gene (PTPN22): Association between a promoter polymorphism and type 1 diabetes in Asian populations. American Journal of Medical Genetics. Part A. 2006;**140**(6):586-593. DOI: 10.1002/ajmg.a.31124

[184] Alswat KA, Nasr A, Al Dubayee MS, et al. The potential role of PTPN-22 C1858T gene polymorphism in the pathogenesis of type 1 diabetes in Saudi population. Immunological Investigations. 2018;**47**(5):521-533. DOI: 10.1080/08820139.2018.1458109

[185] Kahles H, Ramos-Lopez E, Lange B, Zwermann O, Reincke M, Badenhoop K. Sex-specific association of PTPN22 1858T with type 1 diabetes but not with Hashimoto's thyroiditis or Addison's disease in the German population. European Journal of Endocrinology. 2005;**153**(6):895-899. DOI: 10.1530/eje.1.02035

[186] Abdelrahman HM, Sherief LM, Abd Elrahman DM, Alghobashy A, Elsaadani HF, Mohamed RH. The association of PTPN22 (rs2476601) and IL2RA (rs11594656) polymorphisms with T1D in Egyptian children. Human Immunology. 2016;**77**(8):682-686. DOI: 10.1016/j.humimm.2016.06.006

[187] El Fotoh WMMA, El Razek Midan DA, El Shalakany AH. Role of C1858T polymorphism of Lymphoid Tyrosine Phosphatase in Egyptian children and adolescents with type 1. Current Diabetes Reviews. 2018;**10**:2174. DOI: 10.2174/1573399814666180709102533

[188] Haider MZ, Rasoul MA, Al-Mahdi M, Al-Kandari H, Dhaunsi GS. Association of protein tyrosine phosphatase non-receptor type 22 gene functional variant C1858T, HLA-DQ/DR genotypes and autoantibodies with susceptibility to type-1 diabetes mellitus in Kuwaiti Arabs. PLoS One. 2018;**13**(6): e0198652. Published Jun 20, 2018. DOI: 10.1371/journal.pone.0198652

[189] Liu HW, Xu RY, Sun RP, et al. Association of PTPN22 gene polymorphism with type 1 diabetes mellitus in Chinese children and adolescents. Genetics and Molecular Research. 2015;**14**(1):63-68. DOI: 10.4238/2015.January.15.8

[190] Mainardi-Novo DT, Santos AS, Fukui RT, et al. The PTPN22 1858T allele but not variants in the proximal promoter region of IL-21 gene is associated with the susceptibility to type 1 diabetes and the presence of autoantibodies in a Brazilian cohort. Clinical and Experimental Immunology. 2013;**172**(1):16-22. DOI: 10.1111/cei.12030

[191] Tavares NA, Santos MM, Moura R, et al. Association of TNF-α, CTLA4, and PTPN22 polymorphisms with type 1 diabetes and other autoimmune diseases in Brazil. Genetics and Molecular Research. 2015;**14**(4):18936-18944. DOI: 10.4238/2015.December.28.42

[192] Fichna M, Zurawek M, Januszkiewicz-Lewandowska D, Fichna P, Nowak J. PTPN22, PDCD1 and CYP27B1 polymorphisms and susceptibility to type 1 diabetes in Polish patients. International Journal of Immunogenetics. 2010;**37**(5):367-372. DOI: 10.1111/j.1744-313X.2010.00935.x

[193] Pawłowicz M, Filipów R, Krzykowski G, et al. Coincidence of PTPN22 c.1858CC and FCRL3 -169CC genotypes as a biomarker of preserved residual β-cell function in children with type 1 diabetes. Pediatric Diabetes. 2017; **18**(8):696-705. DOI: 10.1111/pedi.12429

[194] Lavrikova EI, Nikitin AG, Seregin IA, et al. Association of the C1858T polymorphism of the PTPN22 gene with type 1 diabetes. Molekuliarnaia Biologiia (Mosk). 2009; **43**(6):1040-1043

[195] Korolija M, Renar IP, Hadzija M, et al. Association of PTPN22 C1858T and CTLA-4 A49G polymorphisms with type 1 diabetes in croatians. Diabetes Research and Clinical Practice. 2009; **86**(3):e54-e57. DOI: 10.1016/j.diabres.2009.09.012

[196] Törn C, Hadley D, Lee HS, et al. Role of type 1 diabetes-associated SNPs on risk of autoantibody positivity in the TEDDY study. Diabetes. 2015;**64**(5): 1818-1829. DOI: 10.2337/db14-1497

[197] Blasetti A, Di Giulio C, Tumini S, et al. Role of the C1858T polymorphism of protein tyrosine phosphatase non-receptor type 22 (PTPN22) in children and adolescents with type 1 diabetes. The Pharmacogenomics Journal. 2017; **17**(2):186-191. DOI: 10.1038/tpj.2016.6

[198] Douroudis K, Prans E, Haller K, et al. Protein tyrosine phosphatase non-receptor type 22 gene variants at position 1858 are associated with type 1 and type 2 diabetes in Estonian population. Tissue Antigens. 2008; **72**(5):425-430. DOI: 10.1111/j.1399-0039.2008.01115.x

[199] Saccucci P, Del Duca E, Rapini N, et al. Association between PTPN22 C1858T and type 1 diabetes: a replication in continental Italy. Tissue

Antigens. 2008;**71**(3):234-237. DOI: 10.1111/j.1399-0039.2007.00987.x

[200] Santiago J, Martinez A, de la Calle H, Fernandez-Arquero M, Figueredo MA, de la Concha E, et al. Susceptibility to type 1 diabetes conferred by the PTPN22 C1858T polymorphism in the Spanish population. BMC Medical Genetics. 2007;**8**:54

[201] Steck AK, Liu SY, McFann K, et al. Association of the PTPN22/LYP gene with type 1 diabetes. Pediatric Diabetes. 2006;**7**(5):274-278. DOI: 10.1111/j.1399-5448.2006.00202.x

[202] Rodríguez A, Alfaro JM, Balthazar V, Pineda TN. Association analysis of PTPN22, CTLA4 and IFIH1 genes with type 1 diabetes in Colombian families. Journal of Diabetes. 2015;**7**(3): 402-410. DOI: 10.1111/1753-0407.12192

[203] Nielsen LB, Pörksen S, Andersen ML, et al. The PTPN22 C1858T gene variant is associated with proinsulin in new-onset type 1 diabetes. BMC Medical Genetics. 2011;**12**:41. DOI: 10.1186/1471-2350-12-41

[204] Xuan C, Lun LM, Zhao JX, et al. PTPN22 gene polymorphism (C1858T) is associated with susceptibility to type 1 diabetes: A meta-analysis of 19,495 cases and 25,341 controls. Annals of Human Genetics. 2013;**77**(3):191-203. DOI: 10.1111/ahg.12016

[205] Wang XF, Chen ZX, Shao YC, et al. Population-based and family-based studies on the protein tyrosine phosphatase non-receptor 22 gene polymorphism and type 1 diabetes: A meta-analysis. Gene. 2013;**517**(2): 191-196. DOI: 10.1016/j.gene.2012.12.076

[206] Lee YH, Song GG. Meta-analysis of the family-based association between the PTPN22 C1858T polymorphism and type 1 diabetes. Molecular Biology Reports. 2013;**40**(1):211-215. DOI: 10.1007/s11033-012-2051-8

[207] Peng H, Zhou M, Xu WD, et al. Association of PTPN22 C1858T polymorphism and type 1 diabetes: A meta-analysis. Immunological Investigations. 2012;**41**(5):484-496. DOI: 10.3109/08820139.2012.664226

[208] Ramu D, Perumal V, Paul SFD. Association of common type 1 and type 2 diabetes gene variants with latent autoimmune diabetes in adults: A meta-analysis. Journal of Diabetes. 2019; **11**(6):484-496. DOI: 10.1111/1753-0407.12879

[209] Dong F, Yang G, Pan HW, et al. The association of PTPN22 rs2476601 polymorphism and CTLA-4 rs231775 polymorphism with LADA risks: A systematic review and meta-analysis. Acta Diabetologica. 2014;**51**(5):691-703. DOI: 10.1007/s00592-014-0613-z

[210] Kumar N, Kaur G, Kanga U, Tandon N, Caillat-Zucman S, Mehra NK. Association of PTPN22 +1858C/T polymorphism with Type 1 diabetes in the North Indian population. International Journal of Immunogenetics. 2014;**41**(4):318-323. DOI: 10.1111/iji.12129

[211] Habib T, Funk A, Rieck M, et al. Altered B cell homeostasis is associated with type I diabetes and carriers of the PTPN22 allelic variant. Journal of Immunology. 2012;**188**(1):487-496. DOI: 10.4049/jimmunol.1102176

[212] Duty JA, Szodoray P, Zheng NY, et al. Functional anergy in a subpopulation of naive B cells from healthy humans that express autoreactive immunoglobulin receptors. The Journal of Experimental Medicine. 2009;**206**(1):139-151. DOI: 10.1084/jem.20080611

[213] Sobolewski P, Maślińska M, Wieczorek M, et al. Systemic

sclerosis—multidisciplinary disease: Clinical features and treatment. Reumatologia. 2019;**57**(4):221-233. DOI: 10.5114/reum.2019.87619

[214] Diaz-Gallo LM, Gourh P, Broen J, et al. Analysis of the influence of PTPN22 gene polymorphisms in systemic sclerosis [published correction appears in Ann Rheum Dis. 2011 Aug;70 (8):1520]. Annals of the Rheumatic Diseases. 2011;**70**(3):454-462. DOI: 10.1136/ard.2010.130138

[215] Agarwal SK, Tan FK, Arnett FC. Genetics and genomic studies in scleroderma (systemic sclerosis). Rheumatic Disease Clinics of North America. 2008;**34**(1):17-v. DOI: 10.1016/j.rdc.2007.10.001

[216] Dieudé P, Guedj M, Wipff J, et al. The PTPN22 620W allele confers susceptibility to systemic sclerosis: findings of a large case-control study of European Caucasians and a meta-analysis. Arthritis and Rheumatism. 2008;**58**(7):2183-2188. DOI: 10.1002/art.23601

[217] Gourh P, Tan FK, Assassi S, et al. Association of the PTPN22 R620W polymorphism with anti-topoisomerase I- and anticentromere antibody-positive systemic sclerosis. Arthritis and Rheumatism. 2006;**54**(12):3945-3953. DOI: 10.1002/art.22196

[218] Wipff J, Allanore Y, Kahan A, et al. Lack of association between the protein tyrosine phosphatase non-receptor 22 (PTPN22)*620W allele and systemic sclerosis in the French Caucasian population. Annals of the Rheumatic Diseases. 2006;**65**(9):1230-1232. DOI: 10.1136/ard.2005.048181

[219] Balada E, Simeón-Aznar CP, Serrano-Acedo S, et al. Lack of association of the PTPN22 gene polymorphism R620W with systemic sclerosis. Clinical and Experimental Rheumatology. 2006;**24**(3):321-324

[220] Burns TM. History of outcome measures for myasthenia gravis. Muscle & Nerve. 2010;**42**(1):5-13. DOI: 10.1002/mus.21713

[221] Xiong X, Xiang M, Cheng X, Huang Y. PTPN22 R620W polymorphism is associated with myasthenia gravis risk: A systematic review and meta-analysis. Medical Science Monitor. 2015;**21**:2567-2571. DOI: 10.12659/MSM.894307

[222] Meriggioli MN, Sanders DB. Autoimmune myasthenia gravis: emerging clinical and biological heterogeneity. Lancet Neurology. 2009; **8**(5):475-490. DOI: 10.1016/S1474-4422 (09)70063-8

[223] Olate S, Muñoz D, Neumann S, Pozzer L, Cavalieri-Pereira L, de Moraes M. A descriptive study of the oral status in subjects with Sjögren's syndrome. International Journal of Clinical and Experimental Medicine. 2014;**7**(4):1140-1144

[224] Wahono CS, Rusmini H, Soelistyoningsih D, et al. Effects of 1,25(OH)2D3 in immune response regulation of systemic lupus erythematosus (SLE) patient with hypovitamin D. International Journal of Clinical and Experimental Medicine. 2014;**7**:22-31

[225] Yuksel S, Pancar Yuksel E, et al. Abnormal nail fold capillaroscopic findings in patients with coronary slow flow phenomenon. International Journal of Clinical and Experimental Medicine. 2014;**7**:1052-1058

[226] Deitiker PR, Oshima M, Smith RG, et al. Association with HLA DQ of early onset myasthenia gravis in Southeast Texas region of the United States. International Journal of Immunogenetics. 2011;**38**:55-62

[227] Nikolic AV, Andric ZP, Simonovic RB, et al. High frequency of

DQB1*05 and absolute absence of DRB1*13 in muscle-specific tyrosine kinase positive myasthenia gravis. European Journal of Neurology. 2015; **22**(1):59-63

[228] Lefvert AK, Zhao Y, Ramanujam R, Yu S, Pirskanen R, Hammarström L. PTPN22 R620W promotes production of anti-AChR autoantibodies and IL-2 in myasthenia gravis. Journal of Neuroimmunology. 2008;**197**(2): 110-113. DOI: 10.1016/j.jneuroim.2008.04.004

[229] Chuang WY, Ströbel P, Belharazem D, et al. The PTPN22gain-of-function+1858T(+) genotypes correlate with low IL-2 expression in thymomas and predispose to myasthenia gravis. Genes and Immunity. 2009;**10**(8):667-672. DOI: 10.1038/gene.2009.64

[230] Gregersen PK, Kosoy R, Lee AT, et al. Risk for myasthenia gravis maps to a (151) Pro→Ala change in TNIP1 and to human leukocyte antigen-B*08. Annals of Neurology. 2012;**72**(6):927-935. DOI: 10.1002/ana.23691

[231] Greve B, Hoffmann P, Illes Z, et al. The autoimmunity-related polymorphism PTPN22 1858C/T is associated with anti-titin antibody-positive myasthenia gravis. Human Immunology. 2009;**70**(7): 540-542. DOI: 10.1016/j.humimm.2009.04.027

[232] Vandiedonck C, Capdevielle C, Giraud M, et al. Association of the PTPN22*R620W polymorphism with autoimmune myasthenia gravis. Annals of Neurology. 2006;**59**(2):404-407. DOI: 10.1002/ana.20751

[233] Provenzano C, Ricciardi R, Scuderi F, et al. PTPN22 and myasthenia gravis: replication in an Italian population and meta-analysis of literature data. Neuromuscular Disorders. 2012;**22**(2):131-138. DOI: 10.1016/j.nmd.2011.09.003

[234] Kaya GA, Coşkun AN, Yılmaz V, et al. The association of PTPN22 R620W polymorphism is stronger with late-onset AChR-myasthenia gravis in Turkey. PLoS One. 2014;**9**(8):e104760. Published Aug 13, 2014. DOI: 10.1371/journal.pone.0104760

[235] Seldin MF, Alkhairy OK, Lee AT, et al. Genome-wide association study of late-onset myasthenia gravis: Confirmation of *TNFRSF11A* and identification of *ZBTB10* and three distinct HLA associations. Molecular Medicine. 2016;**21**(1):769-781. DOI: 10.2119/molmed.2015.00232

[236] Cho SB, Cho S, Bang D. New insights in the clinical understanding of Behçet's disease. Yonsei Medical Journal. 2012;**53**(1):35-42. DOI: 10.3349/ymj.2012.53.1.35

[237] Al-Okaily F, Arfin M, Al-Rashidi S, Al-Balawi M, Al-Asmari A. Inflammation-related cytokine gene polymorphisms in Behçet's disease. Journal of Inflammation Research. 2015; **8**:173-180. DOI: 10.2147/JIR.S89283

[238] Davatchi F, Chams-Davatchi C, Shams H, et al. Behcet's disease: Epidemiology, clinical manifestations, and diagnosis. Expert Review of Clinical Immunology. 2017;**13**(1):57-65. DOI: 10.1080/1744666X.2016.1205486

[239] Kaya Tİ. Genetics of Behçet's disease. Pathology Research International. 2012;**2012**:912589. DOI: 10.1155/2012/912589

[240] Al-Okaily F, Al-Rashidi S, Al-Balawi M, Mustafa M, Arfin M, Al-Asmari A. Genetic association of HLA-A*26, -A*31, and -B*51 with Behcet's disease in Saudi patients. Clinical Medicine Insights: Arthritis and Musculoskeletal Disorders. 2016;**9**: 167-173. DOI: 10.4137/CMAMD.S39879

[241] Baranathan V, Stanford MR, Vaughan RW, et al. The association of the PTPN22 620W polymorphism with

Behcet's disease. Annals of the Rheumatic Diseases. 2007;**66**(11): 1531-1533. DOI: 10.1136/ard.2007.073866

[242] Sahin N, Bicakcigil M, Atagunduz P, Direskeneli H, Saruhan-Direskeneli G. PTPN22 gene polymorphism in Behçet's disease. Tissue Antigens. 2007;**70**(5):432-434. DOI: 10.1111/j.1399-0039.2007.00928.x

[243] Ortiz-Fernández L, Montes-Cano MA, García-Lozano JR, et al. PTPN22 is not associated with Behçet's disease. Study spanning the complete gene region in the Spanish population and meta-analysis of the functional variant R620W. Clinical and Experimental Rheumatology. 2016;**34**(6 Suppl 102): S41-S45

[244] Giudice LC, Kao LC. Endometriosis. Lancet. 2004; **364**(9447):1789-1799. DOI: 10.1016/S0140-6736(04)17403-5

[245] Cramer DW, Missmer SA. The epidemiology of endometriosis. Annals of the New York Academy of Sciences. 2002;**955**:11-406. DOI: 10.1111/j.1749-6632.2002.tb02761.x

[246] Pabalan N, Jarjanazi H, Christofolini DM, Bianco B, Barbosa CP. Association of the protein tyrosine phosphatase non-receptor 22 polymorphism (PTPN22) with endometriosis: A meta-analysis. Einstein (Sao Paulo). 2017;**15**(1):105-111. DOI: 10.1590/S1679-45082017RW3827

[247] Bianco B, André GM, Vilarino FL, et al. The possible role of genetic variants in autoimmune-related genes in the development of endometriosis. Human Immunology. 2012;**73**(3): 306-315. DOI: 10.1016/j. humimm.2011.12.009

[248] Płoski R, Dziunycz P, Kostrzewa G, Roszkowski PI, Barcz E, Zabek J, et al. PTPN22/LYP 1858C>T gene polymorphism and susceptibility to endometriosis in a Polish population. Journal of Reproductive Immunology. 2009;**79**(2):196-200

[249] Vang T, Miletic AV, Bottini N, Mustelin T. Protein tyrosine phosphatase PTPN22 in human autoimmunity. Autoimmunity. 2007; **40**(6):453-461 (Review)

[250] Gregersen PK. Gaining insight into PTPN22 and autoimmunity. Nature Genetics. 2005;**37**(12):1300-1302

[251] Gregersen PK, Lee HS, Batliwalla F, Begovich AB. PTPN22: setting thresholds for autoimmunity. Seminars in Immunology. 2006;**18**(4):214-223. (Review)

[252] Ammendola M, Bottini N, Pietropolli A, Saccucci P, Gloria-Bottini F. Association between PTPN22 and endometriosis. Fertility and Sterility. 2008;**89**(4):993-994. DOI: 10.1016/j.fertnstert.2007.04.008

[253] Gloria-Bottini F, Ammendola M, Saccucci P, Pietropolli A, Magrini A, Bottini E. The association of PTPN22 polymorphism with endometriosis: Effect of genetic and clinical factors. European Journal of Obstetrics, Gynecology, and Reproductive Biology. 2013;**169**(1):60-63

[254] Gloria-Bottini F, Ammendola M, Saccucci P, Neri A, Magrini A, Bottini E. The effect of ACP1, ADA6 and PTPN22 genetic polymorphisms on the association between p53 codon 72 polymorphism and endometriosis. Archives of Gynecology and Obstetrics. 2016;**293**(2):399-402. DOI: 10.1007/s00404-015-3827-6

[255] Gomes FM, Bianco B, Teles JS, Christofolini DM, Souza AM de, Guedes AD, et al. PTPN22 C1858T polymorphism in women with endometriosis. American Journal of Reproductive Immunology. 2010;**63**(3): 227-232

[256] Shi L. Anti-neutrophil cytoplasmic antibody-associated vasculitis: Prevalence, treatment, and outcomes. Rheumatology International. 2017; **37**(11):1779-1788. DOI: 10.1007/s00296-017-3818-y

[257] Willcocks LC, Lyons PA, Rees AJ, Smith KG. The contribution of genetic variation and infection to the pathogenesis of ANCA-associated systemic vasculitis. Arthritis Research & Therapy. 2010;**12**(1):202. DOI: 10.1186/ar2928

[258] Alberici F, Martorana D, Vaglio A. Genetic aspects of anti-neutrophil cytoplasmic antibody-associated vasculitis. Nephrology, Dialysis, Transplantation. 2015;**30**(Suppl 1):i37-i45. DOI: 10.1093/ndt/gfu386

[259] Jagiello P, Aries P, Arning L, et al. The PTPN22 620W allele is a risk factor for Wegener's granulomatosis. Arthritis and Rheumatism. 2005;**52**(12): 4039-4043. DOI: 10.1002/art.21487

[260] Carr EJ, Niederer HA, Williams J, et al. Confirmation of the genetic association of CTLA4 and PTPN22 with ANCA-associated vasculitis. BMC Medical Genetics. 2009;**10**:121. Published Dec 1, 2009. DOI: 10.1186/1471-2350-10-121

[261] Martorana D, Maritati F, Malerba G, et al. PTPN22 R620W polymorphism in the ANCA-associated vasculitides. Rheumatology (Oxford, England). 2012;**51**(5):805-812. DOI: 10.1093/rheumatology/ker446

[262] Cao Y, Liu K, Tian Z, et al. PTPN22 R620W polymorphism and ANCA disease risk in white populations: A metaanalysis. The Journal of Rheumatology. 2015;**42**(2):292-299. DOI: 10.3899/jrheum.131430

[263] González-Gay MA, Pina T. Giant cell arteritis and polymyalgia rheumatica: An update. Current Rheumatology Reports. 2015;**17**(2):6. DOI: 10.1007/s11926-014-0480-1

[264] Stanford SM, Bottini N. PTPN22: The archetypal non-HLA autoimmunity gene. Nature Reviews Rheumatology. 2014;**10**(10):602-611. DOI: 10.1038/nrrheum.2014.109

[265] Serrano A, Márquez A, Mackie SL, et al. Identification of the PTPN22 functional variant R620W as susceptibility genetic factor for giant cell arteritis. Annals of the Rheumatic Diseases. 2013;**72**(11):1882-1886. DOI: 10.1136/annrheumdis-2013-203641

[266] Carmona FD, Mackie SL, Martín JE, et al. A large-scale genetic analysis reveals a strong contribution of the HLA class II region to giant cell arteritis susceptibility. American Journal of Human Genetics. 2015;**96**(4): 565-580. DOI: 10.1016/j.ajhg.2015.02.009

[267] Lester S, Hewitt AW, Ruediger CD, et al. PTPN22 R620W minor allele is a genetic risk factor for giant cell arteritis. RMD Open. 2016;**2**(1):e000246. Published Apr 7, 2016. DOI: 10.1136/rmdopen-2016-000246

[268] Betterle C, Morlin L. Autoimmune Addison's disease. Endocrine Development. 2011;**20**:161-172. DOI: 10.1159/000321239

[269] Skinningsrud B, Husebye ES, Gervin K, et al. Mutation screening of PTPN22: Association of the 1858T-allele with Addison's disease. European Journal of Human Genetics. 2008;**16**(8): 977-982. DOI: 10.1038/ejhg.2008.33

[270] Roycroft M, Fichna M, McDonald D, et al. The tryptophan 620 allele of the lymphoid tyrosine phosphatase (PTPN22) gene predisposes to autoimmune Addison's disease. Clinical Endocrinology. 2009; **70**(3):358-362. DOI: 10.1111/j.1365-2265.2008.03380.x

Chapter 7

Genetic Polymorphism and Alcohol Metabolism

Subodh Kumar Jain, Sapna Sedha and Meeta Mishra

Abstract

Throughout the world, human population experiment with alcohol, result into short- and long-term consequences including increased risk of accidental injuries, risky sexual behavior and lower education attainment. Due to polymorphism in the gene whose product enzymes are responsible for alcohol metabolism, serious health consequences including liver cirrhosis and hepatocarcinoma can occur. Enzyme alcohol dehydrogenase, CYP450 and catalase are alcohol metabolizing enzymes. Polymorphism in any one or all of the enzymes will result in defective alcohol metabolism and acetaldehyde accumulation cause serious health problems. This article mainly focuses on the consequences of alcohol consumption at genetic level that ultimately affect alcohol metabolism resulting in various health disorders.

Keywords: alcohol, alcohol dehydrogenase, cytochrome P450, catalase

1. Introduction

Alcohol abuse and alcoholism represent substantial problems that affect a large portion of individuals throughout the world. More than 200 disease and injury conditions are caused by alcohol consumption due to liver cirrhosis, cancer and various injuries [1]. According to Organization for Economic Cooperation and Development (OECD) report released in May 2015, alcoholism has been increased by about 55% between 1992 and 2012. It is a quickly rising concern among the youth of the country. According to WHO [2], alcohol per capita consumption increased in China and India (China: 4.1, 7.1 and 7.2 liters in 2005, 2010 and 2016 respectively; India: 2.4, 4.3 and 5.7 liters in 2005, 2010 and 2016 respectively). By 2025, the highest increase in per capita alcohol consumption is expected in India and China covering largest population of South-East Asia and Western Pacific region. **Table 1** indicates Indian scenario of alcohol consumption.

Approximately 80% of the college students consume alcohol which can have short- and long-term consequences including increased risk of accidental injury, risky sexual behavior, and lower education attainment. Alcohol use stimulates the Hypothalamic-Pituitary-Adrenal (HPA) axis and causes stress-like cortisol responses [3, 4]. Frequent stimulation of the HPA by alcohol may alter the function of the system, setting the stage for reduced activity to stressors and increased likelihood of alcohol use disorder. Moreover, abnormal stress physiology is related to greater addiction severity, cravings, and poor treatment outcome alcohol use disorder [5]. More than 90% of people who drink heavily develop fatty liver, a type of liver disease. Yet only 20% will go on to develop the more severe alcoholic liver disease and liver cirrhosis [6]. Environmental factors and genetic differences in the

State/UT	Toddy and country liquor (ml)	Beer, imported alcohol, wine (ml)	State/UT	Toddy and country liquor (ml)	Beer, imported alcohol, wine (ml)
Andaman and Nicobar Island	656	532	Lakshadweep	0	0
Andhra Pradesh	561	104	Madhya Pradesh	133	12
Arunachal Pradesh	749	346	Maharashtra	65	19
Assam	304	19	Manipur	155	6
Bihar	266	17	Meghalaya	74	49
Chandigarh	37	42	Mizoram	29	2
Chhattisgarh	120	27	Nagaland	159	23
Dadra and Nagar Haveli	2533	498	Orissa	146	20
Daman and Diu	252	1079	Pondicherry	154	144
Delhi	55	86	Punjab	141	50
Goa	47	108	Rajasthan	80	43
Gujarat	53	3	Sikkim	41	307
Haryana	89	43	Tamil Nadu	20	85
Himachal Pradesh	149	73	Tripura	163	2
Jammu and Kashmir	32	7	Uttar Pradesh	34	5
Jharkhand	320	14	Uttarakhand	38	43
Karnataka	23	102	West Bengal	74	12
Kerala	94	102			

Table 1.
State-wise alcohol consumption per capita per week in India [7].

way alcohol is metabolized, also contribute to the development of alcoholic pancreatitis [8]. Genetic factors, for example, variation in enzyme activity that metabolize alcohol and environmental factors, for example, quantity of alcohol and overall nutrition a person consume play an important role in the etiology of alcoholic liver disorders including liver cancer. It has been reported that in the population of Central India who consume alcohol are at risk for liver disorders due to ALDH2, GSTM1 and GSTT1 gene polymorphism [9, 10].

This article mainly focuses on the consequences of alcohol consumption at genetic level that ultimately affect alcohol metabolism resulting in various health disorders.

2. Alcohol types and components

There are two categories of alcoholic beverages, fermented (beer and wine) and distilled (whiskey, rum, gin, vodka etc.) and the concentration of ethanol differs across preparation. Yeast fermented alcoholic drinks generally contain less concentration of alcohol since yeast stops growing at about 15% ethanol concentration while strong alcoholic drinks/liquors are prepared through distillation [11].

Most alcoholic beverages mainly contain ethanol and water. Some beverages like beer, wine, spirit contain volatile and non-volatile substances along with ethanol. Volatile compounds include hydrocarbons, aliphatic carbon compounds, monocarboxylic acids esters, compounds having sulfur and nitrogen, benzene etc. Dibasic carboxylic acids, tribasic carboxylic acids, coloring agents, inorganic salts polyphenols, tannic acid etc. are the non-volatile substances [12]. Contaminants and toxins found are nitrosamines, mycotoxins, ethyl carbamate, pesticides, thermal processing contaminants, benzene, and inorganic contaminants include lead, cadmium, arsenic, copper, chromium, inorganic anions, and organometals [12].

Regardless of how much a person consume, the body can only metabolize a certain amount of alcohol every hour. That amount varies widely among individuals and depending on liver size and body mass [13]. The effects of alcohol on various tissues depend on blood alcohol concentration (BAC) over time. The time of alcohol absorption, distribution, metabolism and excretion determines BAC [14]. After absorption from small intestine, alcohol reaches liver for metabolism. The rate of BAC rise depends on how quickly alcohol is emptied from the stomach and its metabolism during first pass through stomach and liver [15, 16]. BAC depends on various factors viz. the presence of food in the stomach, alcoholic beverages, the rate of alcohol drinking and genetic polymorphism of alcohol dehydrogenase (ADH) and aldehyde dehydrogenase (ALDH). Depending upon age, diet, alcohol consumption and smoking, the rate of alcohol elimination varies from individual to individual [17].

In the developing world, alcohol use is one of the prevalent habit and is responsible for liver cancer [18–20]. Heavy drinking along with smoking increase the risk of developing cancers [21]. Observations suggest that some people develop cancer even at moderate daily alcohol consumption indicating that alcohol metabolism is genetically determined [22]. Also, those who typically consumed more than two drinks per drinking day were at increased risk of high blood pressure, high triglycerides, increased abdominal girth, and elevated blood glucose. Further, excessive per-occasion consumption is the primary risk factor for both acute and chronic alcohol-related problems [23].

3. Alcohol metabolism

The pharmacologic and potentially pathologic effects of alcohol depend on the concentration of ethanol and its metabolites in the body, and on the duration of exposure to these substances. Alcohol is metabolized in the body by various mechanisms, that is, oxidative pathways involving alcohol dehydrogenase (ADH), aldehyde dehydrogenase (ALDH), cytochrome P450, and catalase enzymes (which either add oxygen or remove hydrogen) and non-oxidative pathways.

4. Oxidative metabolism

Most of the alcohol that people drink is metabolized in the liver. First, alcohol is oxidized to acetaldehyde by alcohol dehydrogenase (ADH). Acetaldehyde is highly toxic to the body, even in low concentrations. In the second step, acetaldehyde is further metabolized by ALDH to acetate and eventually to acetyl CoA, which then is broken down into water and carbon dioxide for easy elimination (**Figure 1**). Thus depending on the nutritional, hormonal, energetic status, the acetyl CoA is converted to CO_2, ketone bodies, fatty acid and Cholesterol [14].

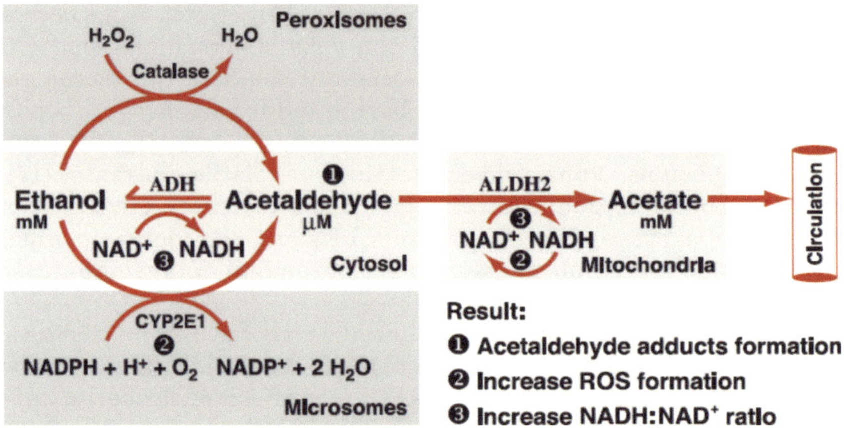

Figure 1.
Oxidative pathway of alcohol metabolism [17].

5. Byproducts of oxidative metabolism

5.1 Acetaldehyde

Acetaldehyde has the power to cause tremendous damage regardless of its short life. This is particularly evident in the liver, where major alcohol metabolism occurs [17]. Minor alcohol metabolism also takes place in the pancreas [24] and the brain, causing damage to cells and tissues [13]. Additionally, small amount of alcohol is metabolized to acetaldehyde in the gastrointestinal tract, exposing it to damaging effects [22]. The International Agency for Research on Cancer [25] asserts that acetaldehyde should be classified as a carcinogen, it promotes cancer in several ways, for example, by interfering with replication of DNA and by inhibiting a process by which the body repairs damaged DNA [22]. Studies have shown that people who are exposed to large amounts of acetaldehyde are at greater risk for developing cancer of the mouth and throat [22].

Acetaldehyde possesses the ability to bind to various proteins like enzymes, microsomal proteins and microtubules. It combines with neurotransmitter dopamine and form salsolinol that cause alcohol dependence and also form DNA adducts, for example, 1,N^2-propanodeoxyguanosine which is carcinogenic [17]. However it is also reported that acetaldehyde concentrations in the brain are not high enough to produce these effects [26]. This is because the brain has a unique blood–brain barrier, which protects it from toxic products circulating in the bloodstream. However, it is possible that due to alcohol metabolism, acetaldehyde is produced in the brain by catalase [27, 28] and CYP2E1 [29].

Acetaldehyde may also be responsible for some of the behavioral and physiological effects previously attributed to alcohol [30]. For example, when acetaldehyde is administered to lab animals, it leads to in-coordination, memory impairment and sleepiness effects often associated with alcohol [26]. Deficiency of aldehyde dehydrogenase (ALDH2) leads to accumulation of acetaldehyde which results in facial flushing or blotches associated with erythema on the face, neck, shoulders, and in some cases, the entire body [31].

5.2 Acetate

Oxidation of acetaldehyde produce acetate which is later oxidized to carbon dioxide (CO_2) in the heart, brain and skeletal muscles. Acetate is also metabolized to acetyl CoA, which is involved in lipid and cholesterol biosynthesis in the mitochondria of peripheral and brain tissues. Acetate causes depression in the central nervous system and also affects various metabolic processes [17].

6. Non-oxidative metabolism

Ethanol is non-oxidatively metabolized by two pathways; first reaction is catalyzed by the enzyme fatty acid ethyl ester (FAEE) synthase leads to the formation of molecules known as FAEEs. In the second pathway, reaction with the enzyme phospholipase D (PLD) results in the formation of a phospholipid known as phosphatidyl ethanol [32]. This pathway is a critical component in cellular communication.

Alcohol metabolism involves both oxidative and non-oxidative inter related pathways. When ethanol oxidation is inhibited through enzyme inhibition, non-oxidative metabolism is increased along with increase in FAEEs in the liver and pancreas [33].

7. The genetics of alcohol metabolism

Alcohol dehydrogenase (ADH) and aldehyde dehydrogenase (ALDH) are the main enzymes of alcohol metabolism. Both the enzymes have several forms encoded by different genes. Enzymes with different characteristics having different ethnic distributions are because of variants of these genes. Since these enzyme variants work efficiently than others suggesting some people can metabolize alcohol more quickly, for example, a fast ADH enzyme or a slow ALDH enzyme may increase acetaldehyde level resulting in deleterious health effects including alcohol dependence [34].

A null allele is a mutant copy of a gene at a locus that completely lack normal function. This can result in to complete absence of the gene product (protein, RNA), or the expression of a non-functional gene product. At the phenotypic level, a null allele is indistinguishable from a deletion of the entire locus [35].

Because of genetic difference in these enzymes, alcohol related problems are either higher or lower in some ethnic groups, for example, *ADH1B*2*, a variant of ADH is common in people of China, Japan and Korea but rare in Europe and Africa [36]. Another version of the ADH enzyme *ADH1B*3*, occurs in 15–25% of African Americans [37]. These enzymes protect against alcoholism [38] by elevating the level of acetaldehyde that make drinking unpleasant [39]. Two variations of the ALDH enzyme, *ALDH1A1*2* and *ALDH1A1*3*, may be associated with alcoholism in African-American people [40].

Along with genetic factors, environmental factors are also important for alcoholism and alcohol-related health problems, for example, alcohol consumption increased from 2.5 to 13% in Japanese alcoholics who carried the protective ADH1B*2 gene [41]. There is no difference in the rate of alcohol metabolism and enzyme pattern between Native Americans and Whites, more Native American people die of alcoholism than any other ethnic group in the United States [42]. This suggests that a rate of alcoholism and alcohol-related problems depends on environmental and genetic factors.

8. Genetic polymorphism

8.1 Alcohol dehydrogenase (ADH)

The major pathway of oxidative metabolism of ethanol in the liver involves ADH present in the cytosol. During oxidation an electron carrier nicotinamide adenine dinucleotide (NAD) is reduced to NADH providing reduced cytosolic environment in the liver cells. Because of byproduct like highly reactive and toxic free radicals and acetaldehyde, the liver cells become more vulnerable to damage [17]. Control of ADH activity is complex and involves: (a) dissociation of the product NADH which is a rate limiting step and (b) product inhibition by NADH and acetaldehyde [14].

ADH comprises of a complex family. In humans on the basis of kinetic and structural properties, enzyme ADH has been categorized into five classes. Most of them are found in liver, stomach and lungs except ADH5 found in most tissues [17]. If alcohol concentration is high, it is eliminated at a higher rate because of high activity of enzymes viz. class II ADH encoded by *ADH4* gene and β3-ADH encoded by *ADH1B*3* gene [43].

Aldehyde dehydrogenase (ALDH2) rapidly metabolizes acetaldehyde (produced by alcohol oxidation) to acetate and NADH. NADH is then oxidized through electron transport chain, or respiratory chain enzymes [17]. Among various isozymes of ALDH, only the cytosolic ALDH1 and the mitochondrial ALDH2 can metabolize acetaldehyde [44, 45].

9. Genetic Polymorphism in ADH and ALDH2

9.1 ADH

Genetic polymorphism in *ADH1B* and *ADH1C* gene locations is associated with different levels of enzyme activity [46]. In different population *ADH1B* occur at different frequencies. For example, in Caucasian and black populations it is predominant, whereas in Chinese, Japanese and in some people of Jewish ancestry *ADH1B*2* frequency is higher. In case of Caucasian populations, *ADH1C*1* and *ADH1C*2* appear with equal frequency [47]. People of Jewish descent carrying the *ADH1B*2* allele show only marginally (<15%) higher alcohol elimination rates compared to people with *ADH1B*1*. Also, African Americans [48] and native Americans with the *ADH1B*3* allele metabolize alcohol at a faster rate than those with *ADH1B*1* [49].

Variants in both ADH and ALDH2 genes can influence alcohol metabolism by either increasing turnover of ethanol to acetaldehyde or deactivating oxidization function of acetaldehyde to harmless acetic acid [34, 50]. This can result in accumulation of acetaldehyde, which is a known mutagen and carcinogen that cause DNA damage and promote esophageal squamous cell carcinoma (ESCC) development [51]. In addition, ADH and ALDH2 alleles may influence individual alcohol consumption habits and risk of alcoholism development.

Information on alcohol consumption, sex, and family history is essential in risk analyses of alcohol-related variants for several reasons. First, alcohol consumption could be a strong confounding variable and effect modifier in comparing genotypes and the risk of ESCC because genotypes and alcohol consumption are interrelated. Second, alcohol-related enzymes do not play a major role in ESCC development among alcohol nondrinkers, or females who drink lesser alcohol than males. Also the adverse role of loss-of-functional *ADH* and ALDH variants will increase in alcohol drinkers. Third, the mechanism of tumorigenesis may not be same with and without a family history of the esophageal cancer [52, 53].

9.2 ALDH

The allelic variants *ALDH2*1* and *ALDH2*2* resulted from genetic polymorphism of *ALDH2* gene is inactive showing no acetaldehyde metabolism *in vitro*.

After alcohol consumption level of acetaldehyde is high in people having heterozygous or homozygous condition for *ALDH2*2* allele [44, 45] and therefore experience negative physiological responses to alcohol.

10. Cytochrome P450

Cytochrome P450 enzymes are present in almost all tissues of the body and play important roles in hormone synthesis and breakdown including estrogen and testosterone, cholesterol synthesis and vitamin D metabolism. Cytochrome P450 enzymes also function to metabolize potentially toxic compounds, for example, drugs and bilirubin, principally in the liver [54]. The cytochrome P450 isozymes, including CYP2E1, 1A2, and 3A4 which are present predominantly in the microsomes or endoplasmic reticulum, also contribute to alcohol oxidation in the liver. However, CYP2E1 is active only after a person consume large amount of alcohol, and catalase metabolizes only a small fraction of alcohol in the body [47]. This enzyme is induced when alcohol concentration is high and it metabolizes alcohol in to acetaldehyde. It also oxidizes alcohol in tissue like brain where ADH activity is low. It produces ROS which increase the risk of tissue damage [17]. When alcohol is metabolized by CYP2E1, highly reactive oxygen containing molecules or reactive oxygen species (ROS) is produced. ROS can damage proteins and DNA or interact with other substances to create carcinogenic compounds [55].

11. Genetic polymorphism in CYP2E1

CYP2E1 enzyme is an important member of the cytochrome P450 family. It is a naturally ethanol-inducible enzyme involved in alcohol metabolism. Polymorphism in *Rsa*I/*Pst*I in the promoter gene region increases transcriptional activity of the gene which may play an important role in the development of esophageal carcinoma [56].

CYP2E1 c1/c1 genotype found at increased risk for gastric cardia cancer (GCC). Individuals with this genotype and have a history of heavy cigarette smoking were at increased risk for GCC. This suggests that the interaction of the *CYP2E1* polymorphism with smoking has a great influence on susceptibility to GCC [57]. Polymorphisms in *CYP2E1* involved in the metabolism of carcinogens tobacco and alcohol, leads to Head and Neck Squamous Cell Carcinoma (HNSCC). Haplotype analysis revealed that haplotype T-A was associated with a greater than 10-fold increase in risk for HNSCC. Use of alcohol or tobacco interact with *CYP2E1* variant genotypes or with *GSTM1* or *XRCC1 and increases the* risk of HNSCC suggest the importance of gene–gene and gene–environment interactions in the development of HNSCC [58].

There was no risk of ESCC found associated with CYP2A6, CYP2E1, GSTM1 polymorphism suggest an opposite role of GSTP1 and GSTT1 polymorphisms for ESCC [59]. Gene polymorphism in GSTM1, GSTT1, GSTP1, CYP1A1 and CYP2E1 represent risk-modifying factors for ethanol related diseases in Brazilian alcoholics and controls with similar ethnic backgrounds. Also the persons with these genotypes are genetically more prone to the development of alcoholic pancreatitis and alcoholic cirrhosis, respectively [60–63].

12. Catalase

Catalase (in peroxisomes) is capable of oxidizing ethanol *in vitro* in the presence of a hydrogen peroxide (H_2O_2) generating system, such as the enzyme complex

NADPH oxidase or the enzyme xanthine oxidase. It converts hydrogen peroxide into water and molecular oxygen. Quantitatively, however, this is considered a minor pathway of alcohol oxidation, except in the fasted state [64].

12.1 Genetic polymorphism in catalase

CAT pathway plays a prominent role in the oxidation of ethanol in the brain [17]. A common polymorphism in the promoter region of the catalase gene CAT c.-262C > T (rs1001179) influences the susceptibility to alcohol dependence and severity of alcohol dependence [65]. It was found that CAT levels were significantly higher in subjects carrying CAT -262 T allele [66, 67]. There is one study showing CAT activity and alcohol intake are interrelated [68], but the impact of this polymorphism in alcohol dependence needs to be investigated for proper conclusions [67].

Author details

Subodh Kumar Jain*, Sapna Sedha and Meeta Mishra
Department of Biotechnology, Dr. Harisingh Gour University, Sagar, India

*Address all correspondence to: subjain@gmail.com

References

[1] World Health Organization (WHO). Global Status Report on Alcohol and Health. Geneva, Switzerland: World Health Organization; 2014. pp. 1-376

[2] World Health Organization (WHO). Global Status Report on Alcohol and Health. Geneva, Switzerland: World Health Organization; 2018. pp. 1-450. ISBN: 978-92-4-156563-9

[3] Gianoulakis C, Dai X, Brown T. Effect of chronic alcohol consumption on the activity of the hypothalamic-pituitary-adrenal axis and pituitary-endorphin as a function of alcohol intake, age, and gender. Alcoholism, Clinical and Experimental Research. 2003;**27**:410-423

[4] Thayer JF, Hall M, Sollers JJ III, Fischer JE. Alcohol use, urinary cortisol, and heart rate variability in apparently healthy men: Evidence for impaired inhibitory control of the HPA axis in heavy drinkers. International Journal of Psychophysiology. 2006;**59**:244-250

[5] Lovallo WR. Cortisol secretion patterns in addiction and addiction risk. International Journal of Psychophysiology. 2006;**59**(3):195-202

[6] McCullough AJ, O'Connor JF. Alcoholic liver disease: Proposed recommendations for the American College of Gastroenterology. American Journal of Gastroenterology. 1998;**93**(11):2022-2036. PMID: 9820369

[7] National Sample Survey Office (NSSO) 68th report on Household Consumption in India in 2011-2012. The Hindu News Report, India

[8] Ammann RW. The natural history of alcoholic chronic pancreatitis. Internal Medicine. 2001;**40**(5):368-375. PMID: 1393404

[9] Mansoori AA, Jain SK. ADH1B, ALDH2, GSTM1 and GSTT1 gene polymorphic frequencies among alcoholics and controls in the Arcadian population of Central India. The Asian Pacific Journal of Cancer Prevention. 2018;**19**(3):725-731

[10] Mansoori AA, Jain SK. Molecular links between alcohol and tobacco induced DNA damage, gene polymorphism and patho-physiological consequences: A systematic review of hepatic carcinogenesis. Asian Pacific Journal of Cancer Prevention. 2015;**16**(12):4803-4812

[11] World Health Organization (WHO). Global Status Report on Alcohol. Geneva: Department of Mental Health and Substance Abuse; 2004. ISBN: 92 4 156272 2

[12] International Agency for Research on Cancer (IARC). Alcohol consumption and ethyl carbamate. IARC Monographs on the Evaluation of Carcinogenic Risks to Humans. 2010;**96**:1-1428

[13] Edenberg HJ. The genetics of alcohol metabolism: Role of alcohol dehydrogenase and aldehyde dehydrogenase variants. Alcohol Research and Health. 2007;**30**(1):5-13

[14] Cederbaum AI. Alcohol metabolism. Clinics in Liver Disease. 2012;**16**(4): 667-685. DOI: 10.1016/j.cld.2012.08.002

[15] Baraona E, Abittan CS, Dohmen K, Moretti M, Pozzato G, Chayes ZW, et al. Gender differences in pharmacokinetics of alcohol. Alcoholism, Clinical and Experimental Research. 2001;**25**(4):502-507

[16] Lee SL, Wang MF, Lee AI, Yin SJ. The metabolic role of human ADH3 functioning as ethanol dehydrogenase. FEBS Letters. 2003;**544**:143-147. http://www.ncbi.nlm.nih.gov/entrez/query.fcgi?db=PubMed&cmd=search&term=12782305. PMID: 12782305

[17] Samir Z. Overview: How is alcohol metabolized by the body? Alcohol Research and Health: The Journal of the National Institute on Alcohol Abuse and Alcoholism. 2006;**29**(4):245-254

[18] Arora D, Marya CM, Menon I. Cross sectional survey on association between alcohol, betel-nut, cigarette consumption and health promoting behavior of industrial workers in Ghaziabad. Asian Pacific Journal of Cancer Prevention. 2015;**16**:139-144

[19] Gao J, Xie L, Yang WS, Zhang W, Gao S, Wang J, et al. Risk factors of hepatocellular carcinoma—Current status and perspectives. Asian Pacific Journal of Cancer Prevention. 2012;**13**:743-752

[20] Hamed MA, Ali SA. Non-viral factors contributing to hepatocellular carcinoma. World Journal of Hepatology. 2013;**5**:311-322. PMID: 23805355

[21] Tong GX, Liang H, Chai J, Cheng J, Feng R, Chen PL, et al. Association of risk of gastric cancer and consumption of tobacco, alcohol and tea in the Chinese population. The Asian Pacific Journal of Cancer Prevention. 2014;**15**:8765-8774

[22] Seitz HK, Becker P. Alcohol metabolism and cancer risk. Alcohol Research and Health. 2007;**30**(1):38-47

[23] O'Keefe JH, Bybee KA, Lavie CJ. Alcohol and cardiovascular health: The razor-sharp double-edged sword. Journal of the American College of Cardiology. 2007;**50**:1009-1014

[24] Vonlaufen A, Wilson JS, Pirola RC, Apte MV. Role of alcohol metabolism in chronic pancreatitis. Alcohol Research and Health. 2007;**30**(1):48-54

[25] International Agency for Research on Cancer (IARC). Re-evaluation of some organic chemicals, hydrazine and hydrogen peroxide. In: Monographs on the Evaluation of the Carcinogenic Risk of Chemicals to Humans. Acetaldehyde No. 77. Lyon, France: IARC; 1999. pp. 319-335

[26] Quertemont E, Didone V. Role of acetaldehyde in mediating the pharmacological and behavioral effects of alcohol. Alcohol Research and Health. 2006;**29**(4):258-265

[27] Aragon CM, Rogan F, Amit Z. Ethanol metabolism in rat brain homogenates by a catalase–H_2O_2 system. Biochemical Pharmacology. 1992;**44**: 93-98. PMID: 1632841

[28] Gill K, Menez JF, Lucas D, Deitrich RA. Enzymatic production of acetaldehyde from ethanol in rat brain tissue. Alcoholism: Clinical and Experimental Research. 1992;**16**: 910-915. PMID: 1443429

[29] Warner M, Gustafsson JA. Effect of ethanol on cytochrome P450 in the rat brain. Proceedings of the National Academy of Sciences of the United States of America. 1994;**91**:1019-1023. PMID: 8302826

[30] Deitrich R, Zimatkin S, Pronko S. Oxidation of ethanol in the brain and its consequences. Alcohol Research and Health. 2006;**29**(4):266-273

[31] Brooks PJ, Enoch MA, Goldman D, Li TK, Yokoyama A. The alcohol flushing response: An unrecognized risk factor for esophageal cancer from alcoholconsumption. PLoS Medicine. 2009;**6**(3):e50. DOI: 10.1371/journal.pmed.1000050. PMC 2659709. PMID: 19320537

[32] Laposata M. Assessment of ethanol intake current tests and new assays on the horizon. American Journal of Clinical Pathology. 1999;**112**:443-450. PMID: 10510667

[33] Werner J, Saghir M, Warshaw AL, Lewandrowski KB, Laposata M,

Iozzo RV, et al. Alcoholic pancreatitis in rats: Injury from nonoxidative metabolites of ethanol. American Journal of Physiology. Gastrointestinal and Liver Physiology. 2002;**283**:G65-G73. PMID: 12065293

[34] Hurley TD, Edenberg HJ, Li TK. Pharmacogenomics of alcoholism. In: Lucinio J, Wong ML, editors. Pharmacogenomics: The Search for Individualized Therapies. Weinheim, Germany: Wiley-VCH; 2002. pp. 417-441

[35] Reszka E, Wasowicz W. Significance of genetic polymorphisms in glutathione S-transferase multigene family and lung cancer risk. International Journal of Occupational Medicine and Environmental Health. 2001;**14**(2):99-113

[36] Oota, H, Pakstis, AJ and Bonne-Tamir B. The evolution and population genetics of the ALDH2 locus: Random genetic drift, selection, and low levels of recombination. Annals of Human Genetics 68(Pt. 2):93-109, 2004. PMID: 15008789

[37] Bosron WF, Li TK. Catalytic properties of human liver alcohol dehydrogenase isoenzymes. Enzyme. 1987;**37**:19-28. PMID: 3569190

[38] Ehlers CL, Gilder DA, Harris L, Carr L. Association of the *ADH2*3* allele with a negative family history of alcoholism in African American young adults. Alcoholism: Clinical and Experimental Research. 2001;**25**:1773-1777. PMID: 11781511

[39] Crabb DW. Ethanol oxidizing enzymes: Roles in alcohol metabolism and alcoholic liver disease. Progress in Liver Diseases. 1995;**13**:151-172. PMID: 9224501

[40] Spence JP, Liang T, Eriksson CJ, Taylor RE, Wall TL, Ehlers CL, et al. Evaluation of aldehyde dehydrogenase 1 promoter polymorphisms identified in human populations. Alcoholism: Clinical and Experimental Research. 2003;**27**:1389-1394. PMID: 14506398

[41] Higuchi S, Matsushita S, Imazeki H, Kinoshita T, Takagi S, Kono H. Aldehyde dehydrogenase genotypes in Japanese alcoholics. Lancet. 1994;**343**:741-742. PMID: 7907720

[42] Bennion LJ, Li TK. Alcohol metabolism in American Indians and whites: Lack of racial differences in metabolic rate and liver alcohol dehydrogenase. New England Journal of Medicine. 1976;**294**:9-13. PMID: 1244489

[43] Bosron WF, Ehrig T, Li TK. Genetic factors in alcohol metabolism and alcoholism. Seminars in Liver Disease. 1993;**13**:126-135. PMID: 8337601

[44] Lu SU, Wang MF, Lin DL, Kao MH, Chen ML, Chiang CH, et al. Ethanol and acetaldehyde metabolism in Chinese with different aldehyde dehydrogenase-2 genotypes. Proceedings of the National Science Council of the Republic of China B. 1995;**19**:129-136. PMID: 7480358

[45] Wall TL, Peterson CM, Peterson KP, Johnson ML, Thomasson HR, Cole M, et al. Alcohol metabolism in Asian-American men with genetic polymorphisms of aldehyde dehydrogenase. Annals of Internal Medicine. 1997;**127**(5):376-379. PMID: 9273829

[46] Agarwal DP. Genetic polymorphisms of alcohol metabolizing enzymes. Pathologie-Biologie (Paris). 2001;**49**:703-709. PMID: 11762132

[47] Lee SL, Chau GY, Yao CT, Wu CW, Yin SJ. Functional assessment of human alcohol dehydrogenase family in ethanol metabolism: Significance of first-pass metabolism. Alcoholism: Clinical and Experimental Research. 2006;**30**:1132-1142. PMID: 16792560

[48] Thomasson HR, Beard JD, Li TK. ADH2 gene polymorphisms are determinants of alcohol pharmacokinetics. Alcoholism: Clinical and Experimental Research. 1995;**19**:1494-1499. PMID: 8749816

[49] Wall TL, Garcia-Andrade C, Thomasson HR, Cole M, Ehlers CL. Alcohol elimination in native American Mission Indians: An investigation of interindividual variation. Alcoholism: Clinical and Experimental Research. 1996;**20**:1159-1164. PMID: 8904964

[50] Birley AJ, James MR, Dickson PA, Montgomery GW, Heath AC, Martin NG, et al. ADH single nucleotide polymorphism associations with alcohol metabolism in vivo. Human Molecular Genetics. 2009;**18**:1533-1542. DOI: 10.1093/hmg/ddp060

[51] Tan SLW, Chadha S, Liu Y, Gabasova E, Perera D, Ahmed K, et al. A class of environmental and endogenous toxins induces BRCA2 haploin sufficiency and genome instability. Cell. 2017;**169**:105-118. e15

[52] Suo C, Yang Y, Ziyu Y, Tiejun Z, Yang X, Tao Q, et al. Alcohol intake interacts with functional genetic polymorphisms of aldehyde dehydrogenase (ALDH2) and alcohol dehydrogenase (ADH) to increase esophageal squamous cell cancer risk. Journal of Thoracic Oncology: Official Publication of the International Association for the Study of Lung Cancer. 2019;**14**(4):712-725. ISSN: 1556-1380

[53] Chen X, Z Yuan ML, Zhang Y, Jin L, Ye W. Poor oral health is associated with an increased risk of esophageal squamous cell carcinoma—A population-based case-control study in China. International Journal of Cancer. 2017;**140**:626-635

[54] Bernhardt R. Cytochromes P450 as versatile biocatalysts. Journal of Biotechnology. 2006;**124**:128-145

[55] Seitz HK, Stickel F. Risk factors and mechanisms of hepatocarcinogenesis with special emphasis on alcohol and oxidative stress. Biological Chemistry. 2006;**387**:349-360. http://www.ncbi.nlm.nih.gov/sites/entrez?Db=PubMed&Cmd=ShowDetailView&TermToSearch=16606331. PMID: 16606331

[56] Leng WD, Zeng XT, Chen YJ, Duan XL, Niu MY, Long RP, et al. Cytochrome P450 2E1 RsaI/PstI polymorphism and risk of esophageal cancer: A meta-analysis of 17 case-control studies. Experimental and Therapeutic Medicine. 2012;**4**:938-948

[57] Cai L, Zheng ZL, Zhang ZF. Cytochrome p450 2E1 polymorphisms and the risk of gastric cardia cancer. World Journal of Gastroenterology. 2005;**11**(12):1867-1871. PMCID: PMC4305893

[58] Ruwali M, Khan AJ, Shah PP, Singh AP, Pant MC, Parmar D. Cytochrome P450 2E1 and head and neck cancer: Interaction with genetic and environmental risk factors. Environmental and Molecular Mutagenesis. 2009;**50**(6):473-482. DOI: 10.1002/em.20488

[59] Rossini A, Rapozo DC, Soares Lima SC, Guimarães DP, Ferreira MA, Teixeira R, et al. Polymorphisms of GSTP1 and GSTT1, but not of CYP2A6, CYP2E1 or GSTM1, modify the risk for esophageal cancer in a western population. Carcinogenesis. 2007;**28**:2537-2542

[60] Burim RV, Canalle R, Martinelli Ade L, Takahashi CS. Polymorphisms in glutathione S-transferases GSTM1, GSTT1 and GSTP1 and cytochromes P450 CYP2E1 and CYP1A1 and susceptibility to cirrhosis or pancreatitis in alcoholics. Mutagenesis. 2004;**19**:291-298

[61] Lakkakula S, Maram R, Munirajan AK, Pathapati RM, Visveswara SB, Lakkakula BV.

Functional PstI/RsaI polymorphisms in the CYP2E1 gene among south Indian populations. Asian Pacific Journal of Cancer Prevention. 2013;**14**:179-182

[62] Malakar M, Devi KR, Phukan RK, Kaur T, Deka M, Puia L, et al. CYP2E1 genetic polymorphism with dietary, tobacco, alcohol habits, *H. pylori* infection status and susceptibility to stomach cancer in Mizoram, India. Asian Pacific Journal of Cancer Prevention. 2014;**15**:8815-8822

[63] Yu BW, Zhang LQ, Teng XL, Zhang Y, Zou LB, Ying HY. Association between the CYP1A1 polymorphisms and hepatocellular carcinoma: A meta-analysis. Genetics and Molecular Research. 2015;**14**:1076-1084

[64] Gropper SS, Smith JL, Groff JL. Advanced Nutrition and Human Metabolism. 5th ed. Belmont, CA: Wadsworth Publishing; 2008

[65] Plemenitas A, Kastelic M, Porcelli S, Serretti A, Makovec MR, Plesnicar BK, et al. Genetic variability in *CYP2E1* and catalase gene among currently and formerly alcohol-dependent male subjects. Alcohol and Alcoholism. 2015;**50**(2):140-145. DOI: 10.1093/alcalc/agu088

[66] Forsberg L, Lyrenas L, de Faire U, Morgenstern R. A common functional C-T substitution polymorphism in the promoter region of the human catalase gene influences transcription factor binding, reporter gene transcription and is correlated to blood catalase levels. Free Radical Biology and Medicine. 2001;**30**:500-505

[67] Hu X, Oroszi G, Chun J, Smith TL, Goldman D, Schuckit MA. An expanded evaluation of the relationship of four alleles to the level of response to alcohol and the alcoholism risk. Alcoholism, Clinical and Experimental Research. 2005;**29**:8-16

[68] Koechling UM, Amit Z, Negrete JC. Family history of alcoholism and the mediation of alcohol intake by catalase: Further evidence for catalase as a marker of the propensity to ingest alcohol. Alcoholism, Clinical and Experimental Research. 1995;**19**:1096-1104